HIV & AIDS

Series Editor: Cara Acred

Volume 314

Independence Educational Publishers

First published by Independence Educational Publishers

The Studio, High Green

Great Shelford

Cambridge CB22 5EG

England

ISBN-13: 978 1 86168 764 7

Printed in Great Britain

Zenith Print Group

Contents

Introduction

HIV & AIDS is Volume 314 in the **ISSUES** series. The aim of the series is to offer current, diverse information about important issues in our world, from a UK perspective.

ABOUT TITLE

Current estimates indicate that there are 36.7 million people globally living with HIV. In 2015, an estimated 101,200 of these people were living in the UK. This book explores current statistics, treatments and medical advances. It looks at the 90-90-90 target set by UNAIDS, which countries look set to achieve this goal and which are struggling. It also considers the ways in which young people are affected by AIDS and HIV and examines the stigma and discrimination that people who are HIV positive continue to face.

OUR SOURCES

Titles in the **ISSUES** series are designed to function as educational resource books, providing a balanced overview of a specific subject.

The information in our books is comprised of facts, articles and opinions from many different sources, including:

⇨ Newspaper reports and opinion pieces

⇨ Website factsheets

⇨ Magazine and journal articles

⇨ Statistics and surveys

⇨ Government reports

⇨ Literature from special interest groups.

A NOTE ON CRITICAL EVALUATION

Because the information reprinted here is from a number of different sources, readers should bear in mind the origin of the text and whether the source is likely to have a particular bias when presenting information (or when conducting their research). It is hoped that, as you read about the many aspects of the issues explored in this book, you will critically evaluate the information presented.

It is important that you decide whether you are being presented with facts or opinions. Does the writer give a biased or unbiased report? If an opinion is being expressed, do you agree with the writer? Is there potential bias to the 'facts' or statistics behind an article?

ASSIGNMENTS

In the back of this book, you will find a selection of assignments designed to help you engage with the articles you have been reading and to explore your own opinions. Some tasks will take longer than others and there is a mixture of design, writing and research-based activities that you can complete alone or in a group.

Useful weblinks

AIDS.gov

www.aidsmap.com

www.avert.org

www.bma.org.uk

www.communitycare.co.uk

www.theconversation.com

www.gov.uk

www.theguardian.com

www.huckmagazine.com

www.huffingtonpost.co.uk

www.ibtimes.co.uk

www.independent.co.uk

www.leftfootforward.org

www.newnownext.com

www.newswire.net

www.royalcentral.co.uk

www.stephenlewisfoundation.org

www.stigmaindexuk.org

www.tht.org.uk

www.unaids.org

www.who.int

FURTHER RESEARCH

At the end of each article we have listed its source and a website that you can visit if you would like to conduct your own research. Please remember to critically evaluate any sources that you consult and consider whether the information you are viewing is accurate and unbiased.

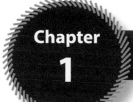
What are HIV and AIDS?

Although they are often mixed up these two words have different meanings. 'HIV' is the name of a virus, whereas 'AIDS' is a name for a collection of illnesses caused by this virus

What is HIV?

HIV stands for 'Human Immuno-deficiency Virus'.

'Immunodeficiency' refers to how this virus weakens a person's immune system, the part of the body that fights off diseases.

HIV has been in humans for many decades but was only identified in the early 80s.

What does the virus do?

Some people notice no symptoms when they are first infected with HIV. But within six weeks of infection most people suffer a short illness (lasting around two weeks) as their body reacts to the virus.

This involves two or more of the following:

⇨   body rash

⇨   sore throat

⇨   fever.

Once this passes an infected person usually feels fine for a number of years.

However, unless they start treatment before the virus causes too much damage, as years go by they will usually start to suffer life-threatening illnesses such as:

⇨   cancer

⇨   tuberculosis (TB)

⇨   pneumonia.

This is because HIV is destroying cells (CD4 or T-cells) that our immune system needs to protect us from infections.

What is AIDS?

AIDS stands for 'acquired immune deficiency syndrome'.

It means a collection of illnesses ('syndrome') caused by a virus people pick up ('acquire') that makes their immune system get weak ('immune deficiency').

You cannot get an AIDS diagnosis unless you are already HIV positive.

In the 1980s and early 1990s HIV treatment wasn't good at fighting the virus and most people with it were eventually diagnosed with AIDS. But now anti-HIV drugs can control (but not completely get rid of) the virus and far fewer people in Britain develop serious HIV-related illnesses.

This means the term 'AIDS' isn't used much by UK doctors now. Instead they talk about late-stage or advanced HIV disease or HIV infection.

What is the difference between HIV and AIDS?

Some people use the terms 'HIV' and 'AIDS' as if they mean the same thing but they don't.

HIV is a virus and people with it have 'HIV infection'. Most of them don't have AIDS.

AIDS is a name to describe a set of illnesses people with HIV eventually get if they don't receive treatment.

But treatment is so good that few people with HIV in the UK now develop AIDS.

There is a test for the virus (an HIV test) but there is no 'AIDS test'.

And people can get HIV but they cannot 'catch AIDS'.

How common is HIV?

Anyone can get HIV, but people from some groups or parts of the world are more likely to be affected. Find out more about HIV in the UK.

How common is HIV in the UK?

Around 101,200 people were living with HIV in the UK at the end of 2015.

Of these 101,200, over 13,156 (one in seven) don't know they have HIV because they have never had an HIV test or they got HIV since their last test.

Recent years have seen around 6,000 people test positive for HIV each year – more than half are gay or bisexual men.

Around 47,000 gay or bisexual men and around 49,500 heterosexuals were estimated to be living with HIV in the UK by the end of 2015.

In the heterosexual population of those living with HIV, 58% are from black African communities.

London has the largest numbers of people living with HIV but numbers are growing in every part of the UK. In the last ten years, the biggest increases in people living with diagnosed HIV have been in Wales, the Midlands and East of England, and the North of England.

Which groups are most affected by HIV?

HIV is largely linked to sexual behaviour: high numbers of sexual partners and anal sex without a condom carry a higher risk than unprotected vaginal sex (which is one of the reasons why gay and bisexual men have high rates of HIV).

People who have moved here from parts of the world where HIV is much more common are another affected group.

HIV infection is also linked to injecting drug use – drug users who share injecting equipment are at a greater risk (which is the reason for high rates of infection in some countries).

Africans and HIV in the UK

Black Africans make up 1.8% of the UK population but 47% of all heterosexual men living with HIV, and 65% of all heterosexual women. Within the African population living with HIV in the UK, around one in nine black African men and one in ten black African women do not know they have it.

Gay and bisexual men and HIV in the UK

Gay and bisexual men in the UK also have high rates of HIV infection.

Nationally, around one in 17 is estimated to be living with HIV. In London as many as one in seven are living with the virus. Rates are even higher among men using the gay scenes of large cities.

In 2015, over 3,320 gay and bisexual men tested HIV positive, a slight drop from the highest ever figure recorded of 3,360 in 2014.

What about HIV from blood transfusions and sharing needles?

Since screening of the nation's blood supply began in 1985, HIV infections from transfusions or other blood products have virtually stopped.

No-one has been infected from a blood transfusion in over ten years. As a result, haemophiliacs no longer have high levels of HIV infection.

In some parts of the world, high HIV rates are found in those who inject drugs and share injecting equipment. Because of needle exchange programmes that give out clean equipment, levels of HIV among people who inject drugs in the UK remain low.

Thanks to antenatal screening programmes, most pregnant women find out about their HIV status and receive HIV medication, so hardly any babies are now born with HIV in this country.

How HIV is transmitted

For someone to get HIV, an infectious fluid like blood or semen has to get inside their body – usually during sex. This can happen if the person with HIV has a detectable viral load and no form of protection is being used.

How is HIV passed on during sex?

During sex, body fluids from someone with HIV can get inside a person who is HIV negative.

If the person with HIV has a detectable viral load, the virus can enter the HIV negative person's bloodstream. This can happen during vaginal and anal sex (and sometimes oral sex too, though this is much less common).

It can also happen when an object (e.g. a sex toy) that has infectious body fluids on it is put inside an HIV negative person.

If someone with HIV is taking HIV medication and has an undetectable viral load they cannot pass on HIV.

Infection can be prevented by using a condom during sex, or by the HIV negative person taking pre-exposure prophylaxis (PrEP).

When is a person with HIV infectious?

Someone with HIV is infectious if they have a detectable viral load.

This is often during the first few months after infection when they have very high levels of the virus in their body fluids and may not yet have been diagnosed.

Early diagnosis means you can start treatment to protect your health and reduce your viral load to undetectable levels.

How HIV treatment stops HIV being passed on

⇨ A person with HIV who is taking treatment and has an undetectable viral load cannot pass on HIV.

⇨ PrEP, when taken correctly, significantly reduces the chances of becoming HIV positive. PrEP is a course of HIV drugs taken by an HIV negative person to lower the chance of infection.

⇨ Post-exposure prophylaxis (PEP), when started in time, can stop HIV infection after sex without a condom (or other exposure) with someone who is infectious – but it does not work every time. PEP is a month-long course of HIV medication taken by an HIV negative person after possible exposure to reduce the chance of getting HIV.

⇨ If a woman is pregnant, HIV medication is part of the way mother-to-baby transmission can be prevented.

Can I get HIV without having sex?

Yes, HIV can also be passed on if you inject drugs and share injecting equipment (needles, syringes, swabs, spoons and other items) that has been used by someone with HIV.

Also, a woman can give birth to a baby who also becomes infected. This could happen during labour but can also take place while breastfeeding or in the womb before the baby is born.

This is now extremely rare in the UK because the following medical interventions can reduce the risk of mother-to-baby transmission to below one per cent:

⇨ the mother taking treatment if she is not already doing so

⇨ she may be offered a Caesarian birth if her viral load is high

⇨ the baby is given a course of antiretroviral treatment for the first few weeks

⇨ the mother is not breastfeeding.

In countries that don't have strict checks on the safety of their blood supply (this began in the UK in 1985), receiving contaminated blood can pass the virus on. This could also happen in countries that don't screen other blood products, organs or sperm.

⇨ The above information is reprinted with kind permission from the Terrence Higgins Trust. Please visit www.tht.org.uk for further information.

Global HIV statistics

⇨ 18.2 million [16.1 million–19.0 million] people were accessing antiretroviral therapy (June 2016)

⇨ 36.7 million [34.0 million–39.8 million] people globally were living with HIV (end 2015)

⇨ 2.1 million [1.8 million–2.4 million] people became newly infected with HIV (end 2015)

⇨ 1.1 million [940,000–1.3 million] people died from AIDS-related illnesses (end 2015)

⇨ 78 million [69.5 million–87.6 million] people have become infected with HIV since the start of the epidemic (end 2015)

⇨ 35 million [29.6 million–40.8 million] people have died from AIDS-related illnesses since the start of the epidemic (end 2015)

People living with HIV

⇨ In 2015, there were 36.7 million [34.0 million–39.8 million] people living with HIV.

People living with HIV accessing antiretroviral therapy

⇨ As of June 2016, 18.2 million [16.1 million–19.0 million] people living with HIV were accessing antiretroviral therapy, up from 15.8 million in June 2015 and 7.5 million in 2010.

⇨ In 2015, around 46% [43–50%] of all people living with HIV had access to treatment.

⇨ In 2015, some 77% [69–86%] of pregnant women living with HIV had access to antiretroviral medicines to prevent transmission of HIV to their babies.

New HIV infections

⇨ Worldwide, 2.1 million [1.8 million–2.4 million] people became newly infected with HIV in 2015.

⇨ New HIV infections among children have declined by 50% since 2010.

⇨ Worldwide, 150,000 [110,000–190,000] children became newly infected with HIV in 2015, down from 290 000 [250,000–350,000] in 2010.

⇨ Since 2010 there have been no declines in new HIV infections among adults.

⇨ Every year since 2010, around 1.9 million [1.9 million–2.2 million] adults have become newly infected with HIV.

AIDS-related deaths

⇨ AIDS-related deaths have fallen by 45% since the peak in 2005.

⇨ In 2015, 1.1 million [940,000–1.3 million] people died from AIDS-related causes worldwide, compared to two million [1.7 million–2.3 million] in 2005.

HIV/tuberculosis

⇨ Tuberculosis-related deaths among people living with HIV have fallen by 32% since 2004.

⇨ Tuberculosis remains the leading cause of death among people living with HIV, accounting for around one in three AIDS-related deaths.

⇨ In 2014, the percentage of identified HIV-positive tuberculosis patients who started or continued on antiretroviral therapy reached 77%.

Investments

⇨ At the end of 2015, US$19 billion was invested in the AIDS response in low- and middle-income countries (not including the countries that have recently transitioned into high-income categories).

⇨ Domestic resources constituted 57% of the total resources for HIV in low- and middle-income countries in 2015.

⇨ Recent updated UNAIDS estimates indicate that US$26.2 billion will be required for the AIDS response in 2020, with US$23.9 billion required in 2030.

November 2016

⇨ The above information is reprinted with kind permission from UNAIDs. Please visit www.unaids.org for further information.

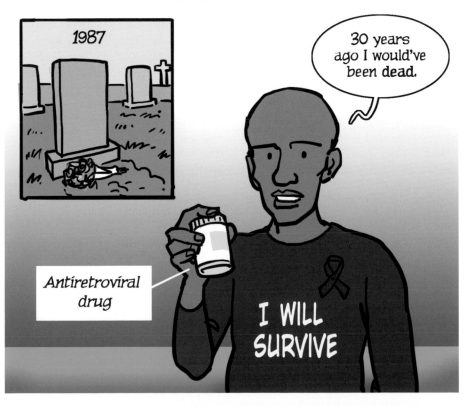

HIV in the UK: 2016 report

An extract from the report by Public Health England.

It is 20 years since the introduction of life-saving, free and effective antiretroviral therapy (ART) in the UK. Treatment has transformed HIV from a fatal infection into a chronic, manageable condition and people living with HIV in the UK can now expect to live into old age if diagnosed promptly. For many people, treatment means one daily tablet with no or few side effects. More recently, it has been demonstrated that the advantages of ART extend beyond personal clinical benefit. It is now widely understood that effective HIV treatment results in an 'undetectable' viral load which is protective from passing on the virus to others [1, 2].

While testing and treatment for HIV in the UK is free and available to all, over 13,000 people living with HIV remain undiagnosed and rates of late diagnosis remain high. Late HIV diagnosis is associated with poorer health outcomes, including premature death [3, 4]. Furthermore, since the vast majority of people diagnosed with HIV are effectively treated, most new HIV infections are passed on from persons unaware of their infection [5]. Condoms remain an important way to prevent HIV and other sexually transmitted infections (STIs) (and unintended pregnancy) and continue to be recommended, with new and casual partners in particular.

Symptoms due to HIV and AIDS may not appear for many years, and people who are unaware of their infection may not feel themselves to be at risk. However, anyone can acquire HIV regardless of age, gender, ethnicity, sexuality or religion and it is essential to challenge assumptions about who is at risk of HIV. As well as increasing awareness of HIV, efforts to reduce stigma and other socio-cultural barriers that prevent people from testing and seeking long-term care must be strengthened.

The good news is that it has never been easier to have an HIV test. Tests are free and anonymous and available at specialised sexual health services nationwide. In most cases the test involves a fingerprick and results are ready within minutes. General practitioners (GPs) and many other healthcare and community settings also offer HIV tests. Alternatively, a blood sample can be taken at home and sent to a local laboratory (self-sampling – kits available online: www.freetesting.hiv) or the test can be performed at home (self-testing).

This report provides the latest data and estimates on the HIV epidemic in the UK and describes the quality of HIV care delivered through specialised services. For the first time, survey data that shows what it is like living with HIV is included, as well as personal quotes to contextualise the experiences of those living with HIV in the UK today.

This report complements an earlier statistical report on the HIV epidemic in the UK, as well as specific reports on HIV testing and on infections, including HIV, in people who inject drugs. [6, 7]. Further information can be found on the Public Health England (PHE) web pages: www.gov.uk/government/collections/hiv-surveillance-data-and-management

Key findings and prevention implications

The number of people unaware of their HIV infection remains high

In 2015, an estimated 101,200 people (95% credible interval (CrI) 97,500–105,700) were living with HIV in the UK, of those, 13,500 (95% CrI 10,200–17,800), or 13% (95% CrI 10–17%) were unaware of their infection and at risk of passing on the virus to others. The majority, 69% (69,500; 95% CrI 66,300-73,700), were men and 31% (31,600; 95% CrI 30,600–32,800) were women[1]. The HIV prevalence in the UK is estimated to be 1.6 per 1,000 population, or 0.16%.

HIV incidence among gay, bisexual and other men who have sex with men remains high

HIV incidence (the number of new infections) among gay, bisexual and other men who have sex with men, hereafter referred to as gay/bisexual men[2], remains consistently high; in England an estimated 2,800 (95% CrI 1,700–4,400) gay/bisexual men acquired HIV in 2015 with the vast majority acquiring the virus within the UK. Overall in 2015, 47,000 (95% CrI 44,200–50,900) gay/bisexual men were estimated to be living with HIV, of whom 5,800 (95% CrI 3,200–9,600), or 12% (95% CrI 7019%) remained undiagnosed.

New diagnosis rates remain high, driven by ongoing transmission and sustained testing

In 2015, 6,095 people were diagnosed with HIV: this represents a new diagnosis rate of 11.4 per 100,000 people. This rate is higher than most other countries in western Europe, the average being 6.3 per 100,000 people in 2015 [8]. The number of people diagnosed each year in the UK has remained around 6,000 for the past five years, reflecting both testing efforts and ongoing transmission of the virus.

The epidemic is diverse

People living with diagnosed HIV in the UK represent a diverse group and assumptions about the characteristics of those living with HIV need to be challenged. Over half (52%; 3,180/6,095[3]) of all people diagnosed in 2015 were born in the UK, compared with 38% (2,820/7,439) of people diagnosed in 2006. This is largely due to fewer diagnoses among heterosexual men and women born abroad, particularly in sub-Saharan Africa; there were 1,110 diagnoses among black African heterosexuals in 2015, compared with 3,170 in 2006. In contrast, the number of gay/bisexual men born abroad has risen; in 2015, two in five gay/bisexual men diagnosed with HIV were born abroad (compared with two in seven in 2006).

Timely diagnosis of HIV remains a major challenge

---

1 Figures presented in text are rounded and may not sum to total, unrounded figures are included in appendices of original document.

2 Gay/bisexual men were previously referred to as men who have sex with men (MSM). The large majority of men who have sex with men who are diagnosed with HIV identify as gay or bisexual.

3 Figures adjusted for missing country of birth information, adjusted and rounded figures are presented throughout.

Fewer people are diagnosed with an AIDS-defining illness or at a late stage of infection (with a CD4 cell count less than 350 cells/mm³), but the numbers diagnosed late remain high. In 2015, among those with CD4 data available, 39% (1,958/4,980) of adults were diagnosed late, a decline from 56% (3,349/5,974) in 2006. Of concern, people diagnosed late continue to have a ten-fold increased risk of death in the first year of diagnosis compared with those diagnosed early. This underscores the need to strengthen the application of testing policies. [7]

HIV care is comprehensive and of a high standard for all

In 2015, 88,769 people received HIV care in the UK, up 73% from a decade ago (51,449 in 2006). This reflects the longer life expectancy conferred by effective ART, as well as consistent numbers of people newly diagnosed. Nearly all (97%) of the 6,095 people diagnosed with HIV in 2015 were linked to specialist HIV care within three months of diagnosis, similar to previous years. Furthermore, the vast majority (94%) of people accessing HIV care in 2015 were receiving ART and as a result have undetectable virus in their blood and body fluids and are very unlikely to pass on their infection to others.

Early diagnosis of HIV infection means better treatment outcomes and reduced risk of passing on the virus to others

In 2015, almost 7,000 people started ART for the first time. This compares with an average of 5,500 each year between 2010 and 2014. This rise reflects revised guidelines from the British HIV Association (BHIVA) and World Health Organization (WHO) [9, 10] which recommend that patients start ART at diagnosis regardless of CD4 count both for clinical benefits and preventing onward transmission. In 2015, two-thirds (66%) of people who started treatment had a CD4 cell count above 350 cells/mm 3 and 41% above 500 cells/mm³. This compares with 22% and 10%, respectively, a decade ago.

How to get an HIV test:

⇨ Go to an open-access STI clinic (some clinics offer 'fast-track' HIV testing) or a community testing site (www.aidsmap.com/hiv-test-finder)

⇨ Ask your GP for an HIV test

⇨ Request a self-sampling kit online (www.freetesting.hiv) or obtain a self-testing kit

Gay, bisexual and other men who have sex with men are advised to test for HIV and other STIs at least annually and every three months if having sex with new or casual partners.

Black African men and women are advised to have an HIV test and a regular HIV and STI screen if having condomless sex with new or casual partners.

References

1. Cohen, M.S., et al., Prevention of HIV-1 infection with early antiretroviral therapy. *N Engl J Med*, 2011. 365(6): p. 493-505.

2. Rodger, A.J., et al., Sexual Activity Without Condoms and Risk of HIV Transmission in Serodifferent Couples When the HIV-Positive Partner Is Using Suppressive Antiretroviral Therapy. *JAMA*, 2016. 316(2): p. 171-81.

3. Brown, A.E., et al., Auditing national HIV guidelines and policies: The United Kingdom CD4 Surveillance Scheme. *Open AIDS J*, 2012. 6: p. 149-55.

4. Croxford, S., et al., Mortality and causes of death among people diagnosed with HIV in the era of highly active antiretroviral therapy compared to the general population: an analysis of a national observational cohort. *The Lancet*, 2016 (in press).

5. Brown, A.E., O.N. Gill, and V.C. Delpech, HIV treatment as prevention among men who have sex with men in the UK: is transmission controlled by universal access to HIV treatment and care? *HIV Med*, 2013. 14(9): p. 563-70.

6. Shooting Up: Infections among people who inject drugs in the UK, 2015. An update: November 2016, Public Health England.

7. HIV testing in England. 2016, Public Health England; Available from: https://www.gov.uk/guidance/hiv-testing.

8. HIV/AIDS surveillance in Europe 2015. European Centre for Disease Prevention and Control; Available from: http://ecdc.europa.eu/en/healthtopics/aids/surveillancereports/Pages/surveillance-reports.aspx.

9. Guideline on when to start antiretroviral therapy and on pre-exposure prophylaxis for HIV. 2015, World Health Organisation.

10. Guidelines for the treatment of HIV-1-positive adults with antiretroviral therapy 2015. (2016 interim update), British HIV Association; Available from: http://bhiva.org/documents/Guidelines/Treatment/2016/treatment-guidelines-2016- interim-update.pdf.

⇨ The above information is reprinted with kind permission from Public Health England. Please visit www.gov.uk for further information.

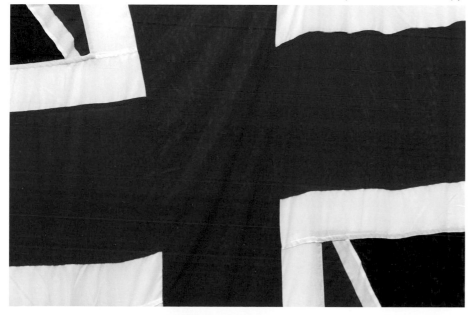

A timeline of HIV/AIDS

AIDS.gov originally posted this timeline in 2011 to highlight milestones of the 30th anniversary of the first reports of what became known as AIDS.

Updated with entries through 2016, the timeline reflects the history of the domestic epidemic from its origins in illness, fear, and death to our present, hope-filled years. Below are highlights from the first point on the timeline (1981) and the last point (2016).

1981

5 June: The US Centers for Disease Control and Prevention (CDC) publish a *Morbidity and Mortality Weekly Report* (MMWR), describing cases of a rare lung infection, Pneumocystis carinii pneumonia (PCP), in five young, previously healthy, gay men in Los Angeles. All the men have other unusual infections as well, indicating that their immune systems are not working; two have already died by the time the report is published. This edition of the MMWR marks the first official reporting of what will become known as the AIDS epidemic.

5–6 June: The Associated Press, *The Los Angeles Times*, and the *San Francisco Chronicle* report on the *MMWR* article. Within days, CDC receives numerous reports of similar cases of PCP and other opportunistic infections among gay men – including reports of a cluster of cases of a rare, and unusually aggressive, cancer, Kaposi's Sarcoma (KS), among a group of gay men in New York and California.

8 June: In response to these reports, CDC establishes the Task Force on Kaposi's Sarcoma and Opportunistic Infections to identify risk factors and to develop a case definition for national surveillance.

3 July: CDC releases another *MMWR* on KS and PCP among 26 gay men in New York and California. On the same day, the *New York Times* publishes an article entitled 'Rare Cancer Seen in 41 Homosexuals.' At this point, the term "gay cancer" enters the public lexicon.

21 September: The nation's first Kaposi's Sarcoma clinic opens at the University of California, San Francisco Medical Center.

10 December: Bobbi Campbell, a San Francisco nurse, becomes the first KS patient to go public. Calling himself the 'KS Poster Boy', Campbell writes a newspaper column on living with 'gay cancer' for the *San Francisco Sentinel*. He also posts photos of his lesions in the window of a local drugstore to alert the community to the disease and encourage people to seek treatment.

By year's end, there is a cumulative total of 270 reported cases of severe immune deficiency among gay men, and 121 of those individuals have died. Some researchers begin calling the condition GRID (Gay-Related Immune Deficiency). This terminology influences both the medical profession and the public to perceive the epidemic as limited to gay men, with serious long-term consequences for women, heterosexual men, haemophiliacs, people who inject drugs, and children.

2016

19 January: The US Centers for Disease Control and Prevention report that only one in five sexually active high school students has been tested for HIV. An estimated 50% of young Americans who are living with HIV do not know they are infected.

28 January: Researchers announce that an international study of over 1,900 patients with HIV who failed to respond to the antiretroviral drug tenofovir – a key HIV treatment medication – indicates that HIV resistance to the medication is becoming increasingly common.

25 February: At the annual Conference on Retroviruses and Opportunistic Infections (CROI), researchers report that a man taking the HIV-prevention pill Truvada® has contracted HIV – marking the first reported infection of someone regularly taking the drug.

3 March: The White House Office of National AIDS Policy, the NIH Office of AIDS Research and the National Institute of Mental Health cohost a meeting to address the issue of HIV stigma: Translating Research to Action: Reducing HIV Stigma to Optimize HIV Outcomes. Participants include researchers, policymakers, legal scholars, faith leaders, advocates, and people living with HIV.

3 March: Pharmacy researchers report finding that women need daily doses of the antiviral medication Truvada® to prevent HIV infection, while men only need two doses per week due to differences in the way the drug accumulates in vaginal, cervical and rectal tissue.

29 March: The U.S. Department of Health & Human Services releases new guidance for state, local, tribal and territorial health departments that will allow them to request permission to use federal funds to support syringe-services programmes (SSPs). The funds can now be used to support a comprehensive set of services, but they cannot be used to purchase sterile needles or syringes for illegal drug injection.

24 May: The National Institutes of Health and partners announce they will launch a large HIV vaccine trial in South Africa in November 2016, pending regulatory approval. This represents the first time since 2009 that the scientific community has embarked on an HIV vaccine clinical trial of this size.

8–10 June: The United Nations holds its 2016 High-Level Meeting on Ending AIDS. UN member states pledge to end the AIDS epidemic by 2030, but the meeting is marked by controversy after more than 50 nations block the participation of groups representing LGBT people from the meeting. The final resolution barely mentions those most at risk for contracting HIV/AIDS: men who have sex with men, sex workers, transgender people and people who inject drugs.

⇨ The above information is reprinted with kind permission from AIDS. gov. Please visit AIDS.gov for further information.

WHO: new HIV cases rise to highest level in Europe

By Agamoni Ghosh

The European Region is battling a record number of newly-diagnosed HIV infections, says a World Health Organization report, with the highest number coming from eastern Europe. The number of new cases diagnosed has more than doubled in the past decade.

In 2014, about 142,197 people were diagnosed with the infection in 50 of the 53 countries of the WHO European Region (includes Russia and other eastern European states), the 'highest ever' since reporting began in the 1980s.

"Despite all the efforts to fight HIV, this year the European Region has reached over 142,000 new HIV infections, the highest number ever. This is a serious concern," said WHO Regional Director for Europe, Zsuzsanna Jakab, in a press release. Data released by the European Centre for Disease Prevention and Control (ECDC) and the WHO indicates that in 2013 there were 136,235 new infections and last year the report listed 142,197 new cases, a 4.4% annual increase.

Of the total number of new cases detected, 77% were diagnosed in the east of the region and 21% in the European Union (EU) and the European Economic Area (EEA). Russia alone accounted for 60% of all diagnoses.

The two biggest concerns in the report, however, are late diagnosis of the infection, and an alarming increase in HIV infections among homosexual men. In the EU/EEA bloc, almost 42% of newly-diagnosed HIV cases were among men who have sex with men in 2014 compared to 2005 when it was 30%. The east in this respect scored quite low with less than 2% cases attributed to homosexuality.

As for late diagnosis, almost two thirds of AIDS diagnoses reported in 2014 occurred at the time of or shortly after the HIV diagnosis. This trend indicates that the immune system of these people had already started to fail by the time their infection got detected. Late detection increases the risks of ill health, death and HIV transmission.

The report goes on to say that contrary to popular belief that migrants may be bringing in the infection, during the past decade, the number of diagnoses of HIV infection in migrants in Europe has declined sharply, and evidence shows that a significant proportion acquire HIV only after arrival in Europe. Jakab also urged countries in Europe to offer HIV prevention, testing and treatment services to all refugees and migrants, irrespective of their legal status.

27 November 2015

⇨ The above information is reprinted with kind permission from the *International Business Times*. Please visit www. ibtimes.co.uk for further information.

© International Business Times 2017

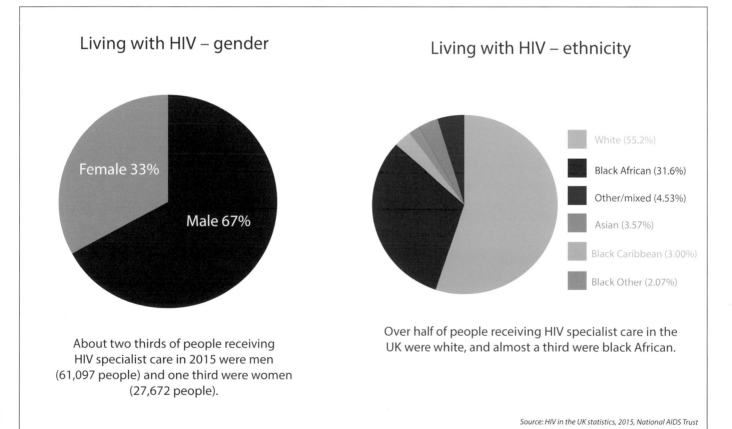

Living with HIV – gender

Female 33%

Male 67%

About two thirds of people receiving HIV specialist care in 2015 were men (61,097 people) and one third were women (27,672 people).

Living with HIV – ethnicity

- White (55.2%)
- Black African (31.6%)
- Other/mixed (4.53%)
- Asian (3.57%)
- Black Caribbean (3.00%)
- Black Other (2.07%)

Over half of people receiving HIV specialist care in the UK were white, and almost a third were black African.

Source: HIV in the UK statistics, 2015, National AIDS Trust

HIV, AIDS and 90-90-90: what is it and why does it matter?

***An article from* The Conversation.**

Glenda Gray, President of the SAMRC and Research Professor, Perinatal HIV Research Unit, University of the Witwatersrand

THE CONVERSATION

Twenty years ago when someone acquired HIV, they would, on average, not live more than 12 years. Today, a young person who becomes infected in the developed world can expect to have a near-normal lifespan with access to lifelong, uninterrupted HIV treatment. Globally, the HIV/AIDS community has worked hard to realise the Sustainable Development Goal of ending the AIDS epidemic by 2030. One crucial part of this plan is bringing HIV treatment to all who need it. The 90-90-90 concept is one part of this plan. Ahead of the 21st International AIDS Conference, Professor Glenda Gray, President of the South African Medical Research Council, explains the importance of 90-90-90 and why there is so much talk around it.

What is 90-90-90?

A concept introduced by the United Nation's programme on HIV/AIDS in 2013, 90-90-90 is a set of goals. The idea is that by 2020, 90% of people who are HIV infected will be diagnosed, 90% of people who are diagnosed will be on antiretroviral treatment and 90% of those who receive antiretrovirals will be virally suppressed. Viral suppression is when a person's viral load – or the amount of virus in an HIV-positive person's blood – is reduced to an undetectable level.

The strategy is an attempt to get the HIV epidemic under control and is based on the principle of universal testing and treating. What is central to 'test and treat' approaches is that if one can identify people early on in their infection, and start treatment so they become virally suppressed, the onward transmission of HIV will be prevented and this will impact on HIV incidence at a population level.

There are an estimated 36.7 million HIV-positive people across the globe. In line with this, the goals would mean that 33.2 million of these people would be diagnosed, 29.5 million would be on antiretrovirals and 26.9 million would have viral suppression.

According to some of the latest figures, there are only 19.8 million people – or 53% – who have been tested. About 13.4 million people remain undiagnosed. There are 17 million people on antiretrovirals while a substantial 12.9 million have not been initiated on antiretrovirals and remain untreated. Of those on antiretroviral treatment, only 11.6 million have viral suppression, which means that almost a third of HIV-infected individuals on treatment are not virally suppressed. This not only impacts on the development of antiretroviral drug resistance and future treatment options, it also has implications for the onward transmission of HIV.

How realistic is this plan?

This is a strategy to try and control the HIV epidemic and get towards an HIV-free world. The concept of universal test and treat is an aspirational concept, but it is an incredibly difficult plan to implement at scale, particularly in resource-poor settings that are heavily burdened with HIV.

This plan entails that the health service identify HIV in people who are not symptomatic, and who are not seeking care. It entails taking HIV testing out of the clinics and into the community, and requires new and innovative ways to get people tested for HIV infection. In order to make this plan realisable, the health system has to endeavour to make HIV testing easily available, even in the most remote areas of the world.

The second component of this plan entails ensuring that HIV-infected individuals are triaged into care, and they need to start antiretroviral treatment as close to diagnosis as possible. People who are asymptomatic and well may not feel ready to start taking treatment for life, which means that there needs to be adequate counselling and support, and the health benefits of early initiation of care need to be adequately explained.

Antiretroviral drugs need to be available in all places at all times. Once treatment is initiated, the aim is to keep people on treatment and adherent so that they can be virally suppressed and incapable of transmitting the virus to sexual partners, and to have maximal health benefits from early initiation of treatment. It also requires countries to have at least three lines of drug therapy. Currently only five countries

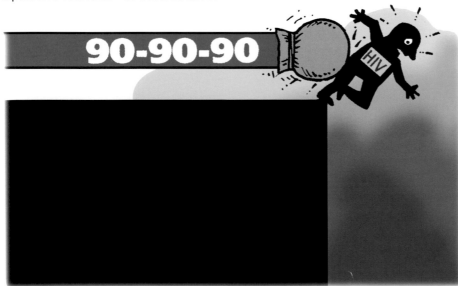

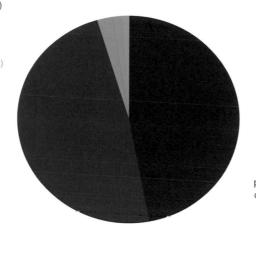

Mode of transmission

- Sex between men (47.1%)
- Heterosexual (48.2%)
- Injecting drug use (2.19%)
- Mother to child (1.59%)
- Blood products (0.87%)

Over 95% of people living with HIV in the UK have acquired HIV through sex without a condom.

People living with HIV who were exposed through heterosexual sex are the largest group, though those exposed through sex between men is a close second.

Of those receiving HIV care in 2015, 41,945 (48%) were exposed through sex between a man and a woman, 41,016 (47%) were exposed through sex between men, 1,909 (2%) were exposed from injecting drug use, 1,383 (less than 2%) were exposed before or shortly after birth and 753 were exposed from blood/receiving blood products. This latter category only included people exposed outside of the UK, as this is no longer a route of transmission within the UK. There are also 1,763 cases which have not been categorised by one of these routes.

Source: HIV in the UK statistics, 2015, National AIDS Trust

in sub-Saharan Africa have three lines of treatment for people to transition onto once they have drug resistance or experience toxicities.

Most countries are unable to realise these ambitious programmes. There are several reasons for this:

First, they require resources for extraordinary access to HIV testing. Second, they need resources to procure drugs and prevent stock-outs. And, lastly, they need resources to keep people on treatment for life. No country either rich or poor can boast this kind of access or resources.

Although resource-rich countries that have less of a burden of disease are more likely to get and retain people on treatment, in heavily burdened countries there are difficult choices to make as a government, as programmes such as this require extraordinary resources.

It entails a robust health system, innovation to improve HIV testing access, and antiretroviral supplies that will be uninterrupted and support all three lines in case of drug resistance. It will entail not only a robust health system but a cadre of healthcare workers who are trained and able to deliver a good service.

It also requires financial investment and a country that sees the investment case and is willing to put its own money and not that of donors into the programme.

Which countries have made remarkable progress towards 90:90:90?

In Africa, Botswana is close to reaching the 90-90-90 target for testing, treatment and viral suppression. Botswana was the first country on the African continent to provide free antiretroviral treatment to people with HIV, starting in 2002. Furthermore, it has achieved its level of coverage when providing treatment to people with CD4 cell counts below 350 cells/mm³, even before moving to providing treatment for everyone diagnosed with HIV infection.

Previous international reviews of treatment cascade performance have shown that northern European countries and Australia have made the greatest progress towards reaching the 90-90-90 target.

At the last International AIDS Conference, it was reported that Switzerland, Australia, the UK, Denmark and The Netherlands were well on their way to achieving this target. In each case, easily attainable improvements in the rate of diagnosis or treatment initiation should allow these countries to reach the goal.

Which countries are struggling to reach the 90:90:90 goals?

Many countries are struggling to reach these targets because of hard-to-reach populations. Testing and treatment has enormous challenges irrespective of the country you live in.

Many of those who receive HIV treatment are those who are the easiest to reach. This means that the road to universal access for all populations still poses major challenges.

There are substantial coverage gaps in many regions. To use Africa as an example: in 2013, treatment coverage on the continent ranged from 41% in eastern and southern Africa to 11% in the Middle East and North Africa.

At least 30 countries in the world account for 89% of all new HIV infections. At least 18 of these countries are in Africa, including Côte d'Ivoire, the Democratic Republic of the Congo, Mozambique, Nigeria and South Africa. But the list also includes other low- and middle-income countries like Brazil, China and India, and high-income countries like the US.

12 July 2016

⇨ The above information is reprinted with kind permission from *The Conversation*. Please visit www.theconversation.com for further information.

Sweden the first country to achieve UNAIDS/WHO 90-90-90 target

By Michael Carter

Sweden has become the first country to achieve the UNAIDS/World Health Organization (WHO) 90-90-90 target, research published in *HIV Medicine* shows. At the end of 2015, 90% of HIV cases in Sweden were diagnosed, 99.8% of people were linked to care and 95% of people taking antiretrovirals for at least six months had a viral load below 50 copies/ml.

"We believe that Sweden is the first country to achieve the UNAIDS/WHO 90-90-90 goal," comment the investigators.

Antiretroviral therapy (ART) has dramatically reduced rates of HIV-related illness and death and the infectiousness of people taking treatment.

For people to benefit fully from treatment they must engage with a multi-step care cascade: diagnosis, linkage to care, engagement with care, initiation of ART and viral suppression.

However, in many settings, even in richer countries, suboptimal levels of engagement with HIV care mean that many people are not benefitting from ART, meaning there are avoidable HIV-related deaths and there continues to be high rates of new infections.

In October 2014, the 90-90-90 treatment goals were launched. These proposed that by 2020, 90% of people with HIV will be diagnosed, 90% of diagnosed people will be in care; 90% of people receiving care will have durable HIV suppression. Achievement of the 90-90-90 targets will mean that at least 73% of all people with HIV have viral suppression, a large enough proportion to have a major impact on rates of HIV-related mortality and new infections.

Investigators from Sweden used nationally collected data to determine the country's progress to achievement of the 90-90-90 target.

Information on people in care was obtained from the Swedish InfCare HIV Cohort Study. By the end of 2015, data on 6,946 diagnosed individuals were included in the study's database.

Surveillance data from the Public Health Agency of Sweden indicated that 90% of people with HIV living in Sweden have been diagnosed.

All new HIV diagnoses are reported to the Public Health Agency by both the testing laboratory and the treating physician. To estimate linkage to care, the investigators reviewed all new HIV diagnoses reported in 2014. Out of 471 cases, 469 were linked to care, meaning that 99.8% of people newly diagnosed with HIV in 2014 were linked to HIV care.

To estimate retention in care, the investigators reviewed 661 people who entered into care in 2013 and 2014. At the end of 2015, 612 of these individuals were still receiving care. Analysis of the people who had apparently dropped out of care indicated that 29 individuals had moved abroad and 11 had died. Nine individuals had no laboratory follow-up in the previous nine months and were therefore considered lost to follow-up. Therefore, 603 of 621 people (97%) were linked and retained in care.

At the end of 2015, 6,605 of the 6,946 people (95%) in the InfCare data were on ART. A total of 6,395 people had been taking ART for at least six months and 95% of these individuals had a viral load below 50 copies/ml. The proportion increased to 98% when 200 copies/ml was used as the cut-off for viral suppression.

"In summary, the UNAIDS/WHO 90-90-90 coverage target of 73% of HIV-infected individuals with undetectable HIV RNA has been achieved, with 90% of all those infected diagnosed, 83% of those infected on ART, and 78% of those infected with a suppressed viral load (< 50 copies/ml)," comment the authors.

They suggest there are several reasons for Sweden's success:

⇨ Small size of the epidemic.

⇨ Legislation that obliges laboratories and clinicians to report new HIV cases and patients to keep follow-up appointments.

⇨ Linkage of patients to specialist treatment centres with multidisciplinary teams.

⇨ Free access to ART.

⇨ High level of adherence to national guidelines by care providers; since 2014, these guidelines have recommended ART for all HIV-positive people.

"We should not be content with these good results, but should continue to improve prevention strategies and increase our efforts to diagnose those still unaware of their infection," conclude the authors.

Reference

Gisslén, M. et al. Sweden, the first country to achieve the Joint United Nations Programme on HIV/AIDS (UNAIDS)/ World Health Organization (WHO) 90-90-90 continuum of HIV care targets. *HIV Medicine*, online edition. DOI: 10.1111/hiv.12431 (2016).

14 September 2016

⇨ The above information is reprinted with kind permission from Aidsmap. Please visit www.aidsmap.com for further information.

AIDS epidemic no longer a public health issue in Australia, but HIV still is

An article from The Conversation.

By Jennifer Power, Senior Research Fellow at Australian Research Centre in Sex, Health and Society, La Trobe University, Melbourne

AIDS is no longer a public health problem in Australia. This is the announcement that came earlier this week from leading scientists at the Kirby and Peter Doherty institutes and the Australian Federation of AIDS Organisations (AFAO).

But what does this really mean? AIDS is the syndrome caused by damage to the body's immune system that results from HIV. AIDS is an advanced stage of HIV infection, occurring when the body no longer has capacity to fight off infections and other illnesses.

However, modern antiretroviral treatment (ART) is so effective at suppressing HIV within a person's body, that people consistently using ART are unlikely to ever develop AIDS.

ART is a lifelong treatment regimen for people living with HIV. If ART is stopped, HIV will rapidly rebound in the body, causing damage to the immune system and increasing the likelihood that the virus can be transmitted to others.

The most recent national HIV surveillance data estimated that 73% of Australians living with HIV are currently using ART. Other research has suggested this figure may be even higher.

Given widespread use of ART in Australia, cases of Aids are so few that they are no longer recorded on public health registers.

This is a major achievement. Since 1982, more than 35,000 Australians have been diagnosed with HIV and around 10,000 have died from AIDS-related illnesses. At the epidemic's peak in the mid-1990s, there were close to 1,000 new diagnoses of AIDS each year – the majority among men in their 20s and 30s.

That Australia can now boast the "end of AIDS" is testament to the internationally recognised success of Australia's response to HIV and AIDS – which has incorporated community, clinical and bio-medical responses to HIV prevention, testing, treatment and care.

But AIDS is different to HIV. While we may not see many cases of AIDS in Australia today, HIV is very much an important public health issue in this country.

There are currently more than 27,000 people living with HIV in Australia and around 1,000 new cases are diagnosed each year.

People living with HIV still require specialised clinical and support services, especially as people age and need to manage HIV alongside other chronic conditions.

HIV prevention is increasingly complex in Australia today. While the majority of new HIV infections still occur among men who have sex with men, we are seeing increasing new diagnoses among Indigenous Australians as well as migrant communities and mobile populations such as transient workers.

Alongside this, HIV prevention initiatives need to adapt to the introduction of new bio-medical prevention technologies such as pre-exposure prophylaxis. Without a sophisticated and flexible approach to HIV prevention, Australia will not be in a position to reduce the current rate of new HIV diagnoses.

Overlaying all of this is the reality that HIV, unlike most other chronic illnesses, is still imbued with widespread stigma, discrimination and misunderstanding.

The psychological and social impact of HIV stigma negatively affects the health and well-being of many people living with HIV in Australia.

One of the benefits to highlighting the end of AIDS is that it draws public attention to the reality of HIV today and how different it is to the 1980s or 90s when AIDS was more prevalent. Most Australians who contract HIV today will never get AIDS. If people have an undetectable amount of HIV in their system, which is often the case among people using ART, they have almost zero chance of transmitting HIV to others.

Much of the discussion and imagery associated with AIDS and AIDS-related illnesses perpetuates the association between HIV, illness and death. This increases stigma, which in turn creates more barriers to HIV prevention, testing and care. So it makes sense to divorce HIV from AIDS in Australia.

But it would not make sense for many other countries. Calling out Australia's success in curtailing AIDS provides a platform to draw attention to other countries where AIDS is still a major public health problem.

Globally, more than 35 million people live with HIV, most of whom live in countries where ART is not readily available or affordable. In 2014 alone, more than 1.2 million people died from AIDS-related illnesses.

If Australia can show that it's technically feasible to "end AIDS", we can see that not achieving this in other countries is a problem of lack of resources and, in some cases, lack of political will, which is often associated with stigma.

Researchers at the Kirby and Peter Doherty institutes, along with AFAO, linked their announcement about the end of Aids to a call for Australia to increase funding to the Global Fund to tackle HIV in the Asia Pacific Region where more than 200,000 people die from AIDS-related illnesses each year.

So there are good reasons for drawing attention to "the end of AIDS" in Australia. But this needs to be read with caution. This is not a call to change Australia's approach to HIV prevention, treatment and care. If anything, it points to the importance of continuing Australia's strong public health response to HIV and for the Australian Government to support a global 'end' to both HIV and AIDS.

12 July 2016

The young people fighting AIDS and big pharma

Demanding radical reforms.

The pharmaceutical industry is broken, and people with HIV and AIDS are dying every day as a result. These young activists are stepping up to lead the fight to fix it.

On Wednesday 9th March, protesters gathered outside a meeting of UN's High Level Panel for Access to Medicines, taking direct action to bring HIV and AIDS necessarily back into the spotlight. These campaigners were from Youth Stop AIDS, a passionate group of young people determined to reform an unjust pharmaceutical system.

In an effort to expose the reckless profiteering of the pharmaceutical industry, activists donned masks of Martin Shkreli, the notorious Pharma bro responsible for jacking up the price of a drug used to treat AIDS-related illnesses by over 5,000%. The masked activists emerged from a makeshift structure representative of 'the system'. The point? That the problem isn't just Shkreli, it's the profit-led system that allows him, and others like him, to flourish.

The action is part of the Youth Stop AIDS 'Missing Medicines' campaign, supported by Restless Development, combining direct action, lobbying, organising locally and awareness raising to expose what they understand as the three key failings of a broken pharmaceutical system.

First, the exorbitantly high prices of new drugs thanks to a lack of competition and restrictive patent laws. Second, the skewed incentives within the system that mean drugs only get produced if they're going to be profitable, not simply because they are needed to save lives. Thirdly, the inefficiency of the pharmaceutical system which prohibits the sharing

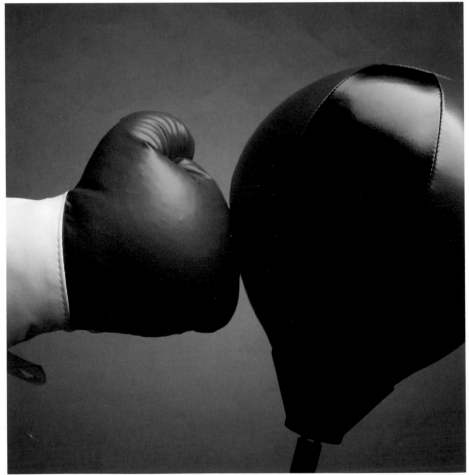

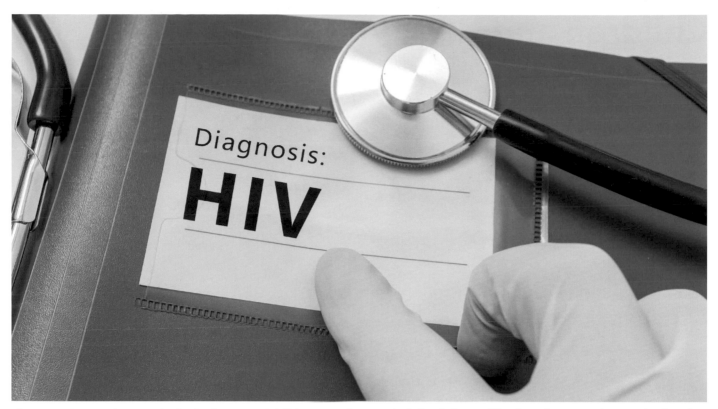

of research, causing projects to be duplicated, and huge sums of money to be thrown down the drain.

Tabitha Ha, Campaigns Coordinator of Youth Stop AIDS, throws those ideas into stark relief: "Treatment costs up to $20,000 per person, per year. Developing countries just can't afford that. Pharmaceutical companies have a hold because they have a patent – they can charge whatever they want because a lack of competition." The system is broken, she argues, and the problem is precisely located with the way research is conducted and funded: "R&D [Research and Development] doesn't produce drugs for those that need them because, often, it isn't profitable. 90% of children living with HIV are in sub-Saharan Africa, millions of them under the age of three. Those demographics can't offer a return on investment, so the companies just don't bother." Her anger at the systemic injustice permeating big pharma is crystal clear as she speaks.

Unlike some direct action organisations, Youth Stop AIDS have what they believe to be solutions to fix the failing system. They are demanding the introduction of alternative incentives and the prioritisation of health research according to need rather than profit. They're also fighting for the

establishment of a pooled fund for research and development, financed by a commitment from nations around the globe to provide 0.01% of their GDP to the fund.

Their aims are ambitious, and amount to nothing short of total reform of the pharmaceutical system, but the activists behind the organisation are fiercely committed to the cause. James Cole, leading up the University of Sussex Youth Stop AIDS branch, cited the flagrant injustice of the system as his reason for getting active. "I grew up with people living with HIV. I know how crucial their access to medicine is," he said. "Internationally, two out of three people with HIV don't have access to treatment. I got involved because I found it completely unjust. It's a denial of everyone's basic human right to live a healthy life."

He was adamant about the importance of youth engagement in fighting the AIDS pandemic: "Transmission [of HIV] disproportionately affects young people, so we need to lead movements to combat it. There's more young people in the world than ever; we need to be at the heart of international development, in every field."

If total reform is required, then Robbie Lawlor, a HIV-positive activist who recently toured the UK speaking about

life after diagnosis, has no doubts that it's young people who are best placed to spearhead the movement. "Young people are a massive inspiration for me because they always want to make change even in the smallest ways. If you engage them by telling our stories, showing the face behind the statistics, they're desperate to make a change." His faith is unwavering: "It never fails."

Ultimately, the activists need the UK Government to radically change tack. Whether it's the swingeing cuts to health services that have left counties such as Oxfordshire without any HIV-specific health services at all, or its reluctance to take on big pharma, the UK needs to change its priorities if change is to be accomplished, argued Tabitha. "I hope that the UK government will put global health needs above profit. At the moment, they just aren't doing that."

9 March 2016

⇨ The above information is reprinted with kind permission from *Huck Magazine*. Please visit www.huckmagazine.com for further information.

Children and HIV & AIDS

Key statistics

⇨ Of the estimated 3.2 million children under the age of 15 living with HIV, approximately 91% reside in sub-Saharan Africa.[1]

⇨ An estimated 220,000 children became newly infected with HIV in 2014, 190,000 of them in sub-Saharan Africa.[2]

⇨ In 2013, approximately 190,000 children died of AIDS-related illnesses.[3]

⇨ Approximately 220,000 children became newly infected with HIV in 2014.[4]

⇨ Between 2005 and 2012, estimated AIDS deaths among adolescents increased by 50%.[5]

⇨ Adolescent girls (15–19) account for approximately two thirds of new HIV infections among adolescents.[6]

Orphans and vulnerable children

⇨ Of the estimated 17 million children who have lost one or both parents to AIDS, 90% reside in sub-Saharan Africa.[7]

⇨ The vast majority of orphans and vulnerable children are cared for by extended family members.[8]

⇨ In some countries in sub-Saharan Africa, 60% of orphans live in grandmother-headed households.[9]

⇨ In a study of ten sub-Saharan African countries, orphans living with their grandparents had better school attendance than those living with other relatives.[10]

⇨ Families and communities bear approximately 90% of the financial cost of responding to the impact of HIV and AIDS on children.[11]

⇨ Children orphaned by AIDS or living with HIV-positive caregivers are at an increased risk of physical and emotional abuse, transactional sex, and HIV exposure.[12]

Prevention and treatment

⇨ Only 22% of HIV-positive children in sub-Saharan Africa who need antiretroviral treatment were receiving it in 2013.[13]

⇨ Without treatment, half of children living with HIV will die before their second birthday.[14]

⇨ An estimated 2.1 million adolescents (aged 10–19 years) are living with HIV, with over 80% of them residing in south and east Africa.[15] Most are unaware of their status.[16]

⇨ In 2013, an estimated 1.5 million women living with HIV gave birth.

85% of pregnant women living with HIV reside in sub-Saharan Africa.[17]

⇨ More than four out of every ten new HIV infections among women are in young women (15-24).[18]

Education

⇨ Each additional year of education dramatically lowers a child's vulnerability to HIV. This is true for girls, in particular.[19]

⇨ According to UNESCO, some 30 million children in sub-Saharan Africa are not enrolled in primary school.[20]

⇨ Children orphaned by AIDS face significant barriers to education, including caregiving responsibilities, stigma and emotional distress.[21]

⇨ The above information is reprinted with kind permission from the Stephen Lewis Foundation. Please visit www.stephenlewisfoundation.org for further information.

1 UNAIDS. (2014) The Gap Report: Children and Pregnant Women Living with HIV. Geneva. p. 4.

2 UNAIDS. (2015). Factsheet 2015: Global Statistics. Geneva. p. 1.

3 UNAIDS. (2014). Children and HIV: Fact Sheet. p. 4.

4 UNAIDS. (2015). Factsheet 2015: Global Statistics. Geneva. p. 1-2

5 UNICEF. (2014). Protection, Care and Support for an AIDS-Free Generation: A Call to Action for ALL children. p. 3.

6 UNICEF. (2014). Protection, Care and Support for an AIDS-Free Generation: A Call to Action for ALL children. p. 2.

7 USAID. (2014). Orphans and Vulnerable Children Affected by HIV and AIDS.

8 UNAIDS. (2015). How AIDS Changed Everything. p. 41.

9 HelpAge International. (2006). Older Women Lead the Response to HIV/AIDS. London.

10 UNICEF. (2006). Africa's Orphaned and Vulnerable Generations: Children Affected by AIDS. New York. p. 16.

11 Richter, L.M., & Desmond, C. (2008). Targeting AIDS Orphans and Child-Headed Households? A Perspective from National Surveys in South Africa, 1995–2005. AIDS Care, 20(9). p. 1019-1028.

12 UNAIDS. (2015). How AIDS Changed Everything. p. 41.

13 World Heath Organization. (2014). Global Update on the Health Sector Response to HIV, 2014. Geneva. p. 55.

14 UNAIDS. (2014). 2014 Progress Report on the Global Plan. Geneva. p. 7-8.

15 . World Health Organization. (2014). Global Update on the Health Sector Response to HIV, 2014. Geneva. p 5

16 World Health Organization. (2014). Global Update on the Health Sector Response to HIV, 2014. Geneva. p. 58.

17. UNAIDS. (2014) The Gap Report: Children and Pregnant Women Living with HIV. Geneva. p. 4-5.

18 UNAIDS. (2014). The Gap Report. Geneva. p. 32.

19 World Health Organization. (2014). Global Update on the Health Sector Response to HIV, 2014. Geneva. p.114.

20. UNESCO, EFAGMR. (2015). Education for All 2000-2015: no countries in sub-Saharan Africa reached global education goals.

21. UNESCO. (2015). Regional overview: Sub-Saharan Africa. Education for all: Global Monitoring Report. p.4.

Young people, HIV and AIDS

Around 2,100 young people and adolescents are infected with HIV every day. In 2013, four million young people aged 15–24 were living with HIV, with 29% aged under 19. AIDS remains the number one killer of adolescents in Africa and the second-leading cause of death among adolescents worldwide.

The majority of young people living with HIV are in low- and middle-income countries, with 85% in sub-Saharan Africa. Countries in this region already have youthful populations, and this trend is expected to increase until 2050. For example, 51% of the population of South Sudan are under the age of 18. For countries like South Sudan that already have a high burden of HIV infections, this will inevitably lead to more HIV transmissions among young people. The number of AIDS-related deaths among adolescents rose by 50% between 2005 and 2012. This is in comparison to a 30% fall among people of all ages living with HIV.

Why are young people vulnerable to HIV?

Young people are vulnerable to HIV at two stages of their lives; the first decade of life when HIV can be transmitted from mother-to-child, and the second decade of life when adolescence brings new vulnerability to HIV.

There is a lack of data showing the proportion of young people infected at each stage, making it difficult to roll out HIV services specific to each group.

HIV transmission in the first decade of life

In 2013, an estimated 240,000 children were infected with HIV from their mother during pregnancy, childbirth or breastfeeding. Many of these children were linked to care as infants, and they need to be supported to adhere to their HIV treatment in adolescence and into adulthood.

This becomes difficult with pressures such as puberty, increased risky behaviours, changes to their HIV treatment needs and new responsibility for their own health. These explain why some young people stop adhering to antiretroviral treatment (ART) correctly during their adolescent years.

HIV transmission in the second decade of life

Unprotected sex is the most common cause of HIV among young people, with sharing infected needles second. Adolescence is often associated with experimentation of risky sexual and drug-related behaviours, increasing a young person's vulnerability to HIV.

For some, this is a result of not having the correct knowledge about HIV and how to prevent it, highlighting the need for HIV and sexual and reproductive health education. For others, it is the result of being forced to have unprotected sex, or to inject drugs.

Whilst programmes to prevent mother-to-child transmission of HIV (PMTCT) have been hugely successful in recent years, reducing new infections among adolescents is more difficult. There are many factors that put young people at an elevated risk of HIV.

Excluded from national plans

Young people are often forgotten in national HIV and AIDS plans which typically focus on adults and children. Consequently, there are a lack of youth-friendly health services.

Data issues

HIV-related data for young people is often divided between adolescents (aged 10–19) and young people (aged 15–24), with less data available for adolescents. However, these age groups are not well defined internationally and even vary within countries, making data collection and its reliability very complex.

Ethical and legal issues make it difficult to conduct studies and research on people under 18, limiting what data is available about how HIV affects young people.

Vulnerability via unprotected sex

⇨ Early sexual debut

The age of sexual debut is rising, showing a positive change in attitudes among young people with regards to sexual behaviour. However, it is still relatively low in many South and East African countries, and lower among adolescent girls than boys in low- and middle-income countries.

⇨ Not using condoms

Condom use among young people and adolescents is usually low, with only 34% of young women and 45% of young men in South and East Africa using them.

⇨ Multiple partners

The number of sexual partners young people have is falling, although it remains high in countries most affected by the HIV epidemic. More than a quarter of young men in Lesotho, Madagascar and Swaziland are thought to be in multiple relationships.

⇨ Older partners

Inter-generational sex (when young people have relationships with older people) is thought to be a driver of the HIV epidemic in sub-Saharan Africa.

Older partners are more likely to be living with HIV, therefore risking exposure to young people. Young women also find it harder to negotiate condom use with older partners who have greater power in the relationship and may use gifts or money to encourage girls to have unprotected sex.

Young people who are part of key populations

Young people may also belong to other key affected populations – such as sex workers, men who have sex with men, people who inject drugs or transgender people. In Asia, 95% of young people diagnosed with HIV fall under at least one of these groups.

These young people are often subjected to strict laws and discrimination relating to their behaviours, preventing them from accessing specific HIV information and services. In some countries, being homosexual, injecting drugs or having sex under the age of consent is criminalised.

Young women

60% of new HIV infections among young people occur in young women, equating to 380,000 every year. More than 5,000 young women and girls, the vast majority of them in southern Africa, acquire HIV every week. In sub-Saharan Africa, women are likely to become HIV-positive five to seven years earlier than men, and girls account for seven in ten new infections among those aged 15–19. Young women aged between 15 and 24 years old in sub-Saharan Africa are twice as likely as young men to be living with HIV.

A number of reasons for this are reported, including gender-based violence and a lack of access to education and healthcare services. In some places, up to 45% of women report that their first sexual experience was forced or against their will.

In many places, intergenerational relationships – between older men and younger women – are also seen to be driving a cycle of infections. Young women and adolescent girls need the means to protect themselves in order to break this cycle. While the rate of new HIV infections among young women in 26 countries is declining, these gains are fragile and by no means universal.

Young sex workers

40% of female sex workers (FSW) in North America, East and South Asia begin selling sex before the age of 18.

In Bangladesh, many start before they reach 12 years old.

The low age of sex work initiation puts young women at an elevated risk of HIV, both biologically, and because of being powerless to negotiate condom use. In Papua New Guinea, 12.1% of young FSW and 14.6% of young male sex workers are living with HIV.

Young transgender people

Data for this demographic is very limited, but one survey in Indonesia reported that HIV prevalence was high among both adolescent transgender people aged 15–19 (5.4%) and young transgender people aged 20–24 (14.2%).

Due to social exclusion, homelessness and financial problems, many transgender people start selling sex at a young age to cope with these issues, which puts them at heightened risk of HIV.

Young men who have sex with men

Men who have sex with men (MSM) are becoming HIV-positive at a younger age. 4.2% of young MSM under 25 are living with HIV, compared to 3.7% among all MSM.

In Bangkok, Thailand, HIV incidence among young MSM has risen dramatically, from 4.1% in 2003 to 25% in 2012.

Young people who inject drugs

HIV prevalence among young people who inject drugs worldwide is 5.2%. However, it is much higher in countries such as Pakistan, where 23% of young people aged 15–24 who inject drugs are living with HIV.

Many drug users who start injecting young are more likely to become HIV-positive because they are:

⇨ less likely to access harm reduction and treatment services

⇨ more likely to share needles and syringes

⇨ more likely to rely on older drug users for equipment

⇨ less likely to understand the risks of injecting

⇨ likely to require parental consent to access HIV testing, needles from pharmacies and harm reduction programmes.

There are often age restrictions on accessing harm reduction services, forcing young people away from services and being denied help to overcome their addiction. If someone starts injecting drugs in their youth, they should be prioritised for harm reduction services, not denied them.

HIV prevention programmes for young people

Age-appropriate services

Young people respond much better to HIV and sexual health services that are specific to their age group. This includes sexual and reproductive health education, contraception and condoms, mental health services, peer support, and support transferring from paediatric to adult health services.

Greater emphasis should be placed on counselling to encourage behaviour change among young people, rather than just handing out commodities such as condoms.

Voluntary medical male circumcision (VMMC)

The effect of male circumcision on reducing transmission of HIV from

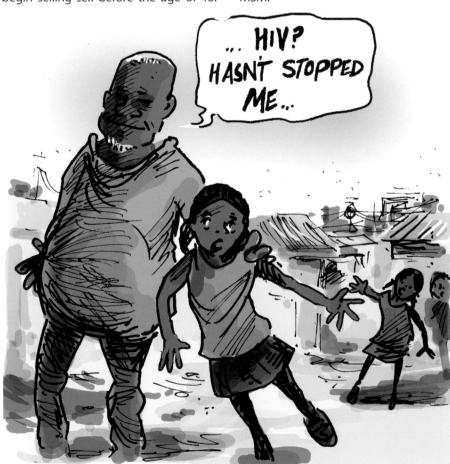

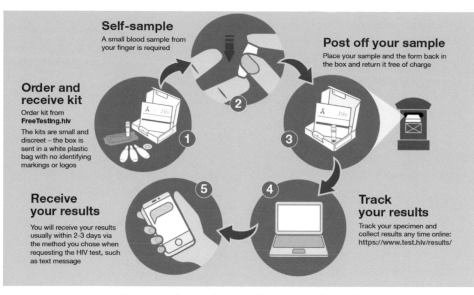

Self-sample
A small blood sample from your finger is required

Post off your sample
Place your sample and the form back in the box and return it free of charge

Order and receive kit
Order kit from **FreeTesting.hiv**
The kits are small and discreet – the box is sent in a white plastic bag with no identifying markings or logos

Track your results
Track your specimen and collect results any time online: https://www.test.hiv/results/

Receive your results
You will receive your results usually within 2-3 days via the method you chose when requesting the HIV test, such as text message

women to men via vaginal sex has shown to be most successful among men under the age of 25. This is likely due to the fact that it is easier to encourage safer sexual behaviour among younger people than older people who have already established behavioural norms.

Younger males also face less pressure from female partners when abstaining from sex during the healing process, due to greater cultural acceptance of circumcision among younger people.

Engaging schools in the response

Schools have the potential to provide detailed education on HIV and AIDS and other sexual health issues. More progress needs to be made to ensure there is equality in access to schools by both girls and boys, and to prevent them from dropping out.

Engaging young people in the response

Young people have the potential to be great peer educators, and to help in the design of HIV-related services and programmes. Technology and social media are consistently being proved as effective ways to engage young people in sharing HIV knowledge.

These peer educator and social media ideas have been combined by the Y+ Programme, a platform for young people living with HIV to talk, find a mentor, become a mentor and advocate for the needs of young people.

Cash transfers plus care

Small cash transfers to households on a very low income have been shown to have a positive effect on reducing risk-taking behaviour among adolescent girls in South Africa. The study also found that HIV incidence halved among both girls and boys who received cash, coupled with other forms of care, known as 'cash plus care'.

HIV testing and counselling (HTC) for young people

It's thought that only 10% of young men and 15% of young women living in sub-Saharan Africa know their HIV status.

Increasing access to HIV testing is vital to prevent further transmission of HIV among young people. Mobile and community testing initiatives are a successful way of reaching young people who are less likely to voluntarily visit a static testing centre. HTC has proved very successful as a form of HIV prevention in Eastern and Southern Africa. A study in South Africa found that HIV testing and counselling (HTC) among 4,000 young people caused 41% fewer cases of HIV transmission in a four-year period.

Barriers to HIV testing for young people

The World Health Organization (WHO) 2013 guidelines for HIV testing and counselling for adolescents highlight the programmatic barriers currently preventing adolescents from accessing HIV testing, and what can be done to overcome them.

⇨ Age of consent to HIV testing

In many countries, the age of consent is high at around 18–21, leaving people younger than this having to obtain parental consent. This is much more likely to result in a young person not getting an HIV test when discussions with parents around sexual relations and HIV are necessary.

For many orphaned young people, parental consent is not an option and so they are denied access. Age of consent laws to HIV testing should be removed.

⇨ Age-appropriate HTC

Services must be open at appropriate times (after school/college), and be at appropriate venues where young people feel safe enough to go alone.

⇨ Legal protection

In the case of sexual violence, it is important that a young person is supported and referred to child protection services.

⇨ Linking to treatment and care

Young people need extra support to transfer to treatment if they test positive, as they may otherwise get lost in the treatment cascade.

⇨ Support around disclosure

Due to common low ages of sexual debut and age of first childbirth, it is important that young people are supported to protect the health of their partner(s) through disclosure.

Antiretroviral treatment for young people

Mother-to-child transmission (MTCT) rates are decreasing, but the fact that it still exists means that there will be an increase in adolescents needing antiretroviral treatment (ART) until it is eliminated. Access to ART for young people is unknown because data is disaggregated into children under 15 years and adults over 15 years.

For those who do access treatment, there are some common barriers to its effectiveness.

Adhering to antiretroviral treatment

Adherence to ART among young people has increased since 2005, thought to be due to more manageable antiretroviral drugs (ARV), less toxicity, and combined treatment. However, adherence support must be scaled up for young people to sustain treatment as a form of prevention, and stop onwards transmission to others.

Treatment adherence is greatest in Africa and Asia (84%), and lowest in North America (53%). One reason for this difference is the variation in ages of maturation. It is generally thought that young people mature earlier in Africa and Asia, where they start working and have relationships at a younger age. This bears great responsibilities, which may contribute to young people being more responsible for their own healthcare, and adhering to their treatment.

Transitioning from paediatric to adult care

In North America and Europe, there is a large jump at 18 years of age, when people living with HIV are moved from paediatric to adult services and allocated a new doctor.

This transition is complicated by the added pressure of suddenly becoming responsible for their own lifelong treatment rather than with support from guardians. At this point, a lot of young people are lost to follow up and no longer retained in care.

Increased drug doses

Changing ARV regimens and doses during adolescence is another complex issue that results in young people not adhering to their treatment. As young people grow, their dosages must be increased to reflect increases in their weight and height.

Lost from the treatment system

One study that took place in clinics in Kenya, Mozambique, Tanzania and Rwanda found that young people were more likely to be lost from treatment services than older people. Clinics that offer condoms and youth support groups experienced greater retention in care, showing that youth-friendly services ensure young patients are retained in care.

Barriers to HIV prevention among young people

Low HIV and sexual health knowledge

In East and South African countries, only 40% of young people know how to prevent HIV because sex education in these countries is low.

Only 36% of young men and 28% of young women in sub-Saharan Africa have accurate HIV knowledge. This is unsurprising in a region where many children drop out of primary school and only 20% complete secondary school.

Opportunities to obtain knowledge about HIV, AIDS and sexual health are extremely limited for young people not in school. Youth clubs have the potential to provide HIV knowledge, but their small, localised reach means their impact is limited on a large scale.

Lack of access to HIV services

Many young people report that healthcare workers have negative attitudes towards young people seeking healthcare services, particularly those having sex under the national age of consent, engaging in homosexual relationships or using drugs. This deters them from seeking contraception, sexually transmitted infection (STI) check-ups and HIV testing.

Some young people are also fearful of stigma from their partners, families and communities, making them unwilling to come forward for HIV testing in case their families find out that they are sexually active or living with HIV. Other sexual and reproductive health services deny access to people who are not married.

Gender inequality and HIV vulnerability

Of all adolescents aged 15-19 who were diagnosed as HIV-positive during 2012, two-thirds were girls. Globally, young girls are more vulnerable to HIV for a number of reasons, but universally the level of HIV knowledge among girls is less than among boys because girls are less likely to attend and finish secondary school.

In order to address these gender differences, a systematic review of HIV programming for adolescents noted a number of interventions that are needed for programmes to be effective for girls:

⇨ an enabling environment, including keeping girls in school, promoting gender equity, strengthening protective legal norms, and reducing gender-based violence

⇨ information and service needs, including provision of age-appropriate comprehensive sex education, increasing knowledge

about and access to information and services, and expanding harm reduction programs for adolescent girls who inject drugs

⇨ social support, including promoting caring relationships with adults and providing support for adolescent female orphans and vulnerable children.

Young parenthood and HIV

15 million girls between 15 and 19 give birth every year. In certain countries, the average age of parenthood is even lower – 41% of girls in Sierra Leone have their first pregnancy between 12 and 14 years of age.

As a result, young women are more likely to learn their HIV status before their partner does via antenatal clinic tests. This generates a culture of blame on the woman because she found out first, reducing her willingness to seek future healthcare services.

The future of HIV among young people

Among young people, the age of sexual debut is rising, the number of sexual partners is falling and the uptake of voluntary medical male circumcision is most popular among people younger than 25.

Still, young people are routinely forgotten in national strategic plans to tackle the HIV epidemic, especially those that also fall under other key affected populations. They are not targeted with age-appropriate HIV prevention programmes and data about their vulnerability is not collected.

As a result, young people are often forgotten and excluded from the international HIV response. Engaging young people is key to protecting their health and addressing the HIV epidemic as a whole.

For full references see: https://www.avert. org/professionals/hiv-social-issues/key-affected-populations/young-people.

2 February 2017

⇨ The above information is reprinted with kind permission from AVERT. Please visit www.avert.org for further information.

How schools are getting it wrong on HIV and AIDS

Children have been humiliated in school and even excluded because many teachers are still badly informed.

By Joanna Moorhead

Leo found out he was HIV positive when he was 12. A few months later, in a personal, social and health education lesson, the teacher was discussing HIV and AIDS: "And some of the pupils were joking around, and the teacher said: 'Guys, it's not funny! If you have HIV, you don't have long to live. If you have HIV, you're going to die.'"

Leo remembers trying to remain composed, but he couldn't: what he'd heard was so shocking, so unexpected. His teacher noticed the tears running down his face, took him out of the classroom and asked: "What's wrong?" And Leo said: "Is that what's going to happen to me, sir? I'm HIV positive."

The truth is that Leo isn't, and never was, going to die. Like most of the 1,000 or so school-age children in the UK who are HIV positive, his condition is carefully monitored and well managed by drugs. What he heard from his teacher that day was incorrect: misinformation from someone in a trusted position who a pupil would usually expect to be correct.

Leo's tale is one of many examples of how wrong schools often get it where HIV is concerned. Students have been humiliated and shocked in their own schools, and some are reported to have been excluded by their school on disclosure of their HIV status.

As well as causing distress to affected pupils, teachers' misconceptions – when passed on to other children – ensure a new generation is, in turn, misinformed. All of which explains why the Children's HIV Association (Chiva) is reissuing guidelines for schools this week, and why its projects manager, Magda Conway, says all teachers need to become much more aware of the issues around pupils who are HIV positive or who are affected by HIV through someone close to them. "Teachers aren't a bad lot, we don't want to vilify them, but many of them are very ill informed about this," says Conway. One survey carried out by Chiva last year found that fewer than half of teachers were aware that mother-to-child transmission is the most common route of infection to children, and more than 50% believed HIV could be transmitted via spitting or biting

"The problem is that many of them got their information about HIV from the notorious AIDS campaign of the 1980s – the 'Don't die of ignorance' campaign," says Conway. That campaign, run at saturation levels by the Department of Health, featured crumbling mountains and a falling tombstone, and a voiceover that spoke of the virus as "a threat to us all", the cause of "a deadly disease [with] no known cure".

"Science has come on in leaps and bounds since then – today it's a manageable health condition, and it needs to be treated that way. Too many teachers still base what they know on the 'Don't die of ignorance' campaign."

She says schools need to ensure that a pupil who discloses their HIV diagnosis will be sensitively and professionally supported. "If teachers become aware that a child in school is living with HIV, they need to understand that there is no risk to anyone else, and that confidentiality should be respected." The revised guidelines spell out the most misunderstood key facts, including the crucial issue that HIV cannot be passed on through normal play and normal childhood interactions.

"No one has ever contracted HIV in school, period," says Conway. "A pupil or a teacher living with HIV poses no risk whatsoever to the school community."

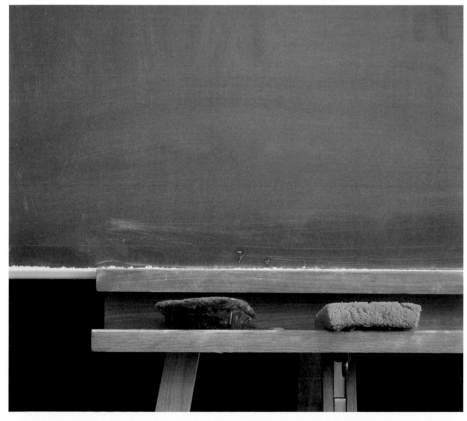

Those with HIV, the guidelines spell out, can have every expectation of living long and happy lives. And confidentiality is essential to people living with HIV, due to the stigma that remains in society around the virus.

In an attempt to step up awareness, Chiva took Leo and a group of other HIV-positive young people to a meeting at Westminster last week, where they shared their stories with MPs and peers.

Cece, 17, told how her boyfriend found out she was HIV positive and started spreading the story around the school. "I stopped taking my meds because I thought that would be a way of forgetting about it – everything seemed so awful," she says. "When you're HIV positive you live a double life, and at some point it's going to cross over." And what happened next? "You really find out who your friends are: a group of my friends got the kids together who knew and said, stop spreading these stories. But the point is that it should have been the teachers who did that, not the children."

Sometimes the ignorance of teachers puts their better-informed pupils into a difficult situation, as happened to another pupil, Evie. "We were in a science lesson and the teacher was asked, how is the HIV virus passed on? And the teacher said, you can get it from kissing someone. And I knew, of course, that this wasn't true, but I wasn't able to put the teacher right because how could I have explained how I knew without disclosing my own HIV status, which it wouldn't have been appropriate to do?"

As heartbreaking as Leo's experience was that of Shona, who, like Leo,

knew she was HIV positive but hadn't disclosed it to her school. "I was in a humanities class and the teacher started going on about what HIV meant. She said if you have it, your life expectancy is probably going to be about ten years. And I was in year nine so about 13 at the time, and it was shocking and confusing. I thought, does that mean I'll only live another 10 years? It wasn't what I'd been told, but when you hear a teacher saying something like that, it makes you doubt what you thought you knew."

Other youngsters told stories about overreaction on the part of their teachers when their status was disclosed. One boy talked of feeling alarm bells were ringing when he had a nose bleed; a girl spoke about how she was offered a nurse to talk to daily. "I said, I don't need to talk to a nurse every day! I see enough nurses. I just want a normal life."

The lack of good management for HIV-positive pupils means they sometimes miss out on, for example, school trips – as happened to Cece. "I wanted to go on a skiing trip to Austria when I was in year eight. It was ten days away, and as soon as I told my mum she was like, how on earth can you do that? You have to take your medicines, you can't go abroad." Cece didn't go on the trip. "But why should I have missed out? The truth is I could easily have gone on that trip if there had been proper support for me in the school."

What schools need to provide, says Conway, is the potential for a pupil who is HIV positive to tell one trusted person. "You get some schools where it's discovered that a pupil is HIV positive and there's a kneejerk

reaction based on ignorance. I've heard of pupils even being excluded – that happened as recently as 2013," says Conway. In that instance it was a third party, a community worker, who disclosed the pupil's HIV status to the school, which then took advice from a national teaching organisation – advice that turned out to be 25 years out of date. At another school she was told about, says Conway, the headteacher told an assembly that a pupil was HIV positive and was being excluded.

The National Association of Head Teachers is backing the Chiva campaign. Its president, Tony Draper, says schools need to make themselves safe places for children who are HIV positive. "They need to ensure that pupils can disclose their status to one person, and no one else needs to know," he says. "At the moment, pupils are missing school for medical appointments without being able to tell anyone why they're away. That needs to change."

The truth is, says Conway, that the treatment of pupils with HIV should be the same as the treatment for any other pupil: there are no special requirements, except the need for one person they can feel confident in disclosing their status to, should they choose to. "The biggest thing we're fighting is the stigma that surrounds HIV, and the biggest problem for pupils who live with HIV isn't physical health issues, it's mental health issues. Children who are HIV positive are more likely to have mental health problems, more likely to self-harm, and more likely to take their own lives. And that's all connected to the pressures that go with being HIV positive – and that's what we want schools to help change."

All children's names have been changed.

25 November 2015

⇨ The above information is reprinted with kind permission from *The Guardian*. Please visit www.theguardian.com for further information.

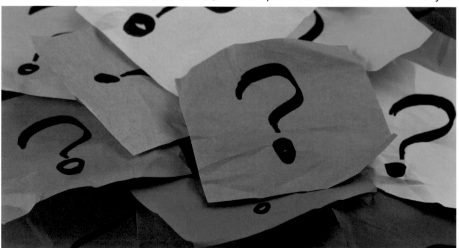

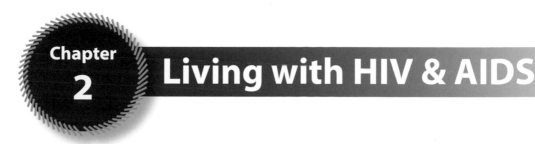
HIV Stigma Survey, UK 2015

HIV testing, diagnosis and treatment

Nine in ten participants had first been diagnosed with HIV in the UK. Over two thirds of these were diagnosed more than five years ago and 9% were diagnosed in the previous year (this is comparable to UK-wide surveillance data). The large majority of those diagnosed in the last five years in the UK reported being tested voluntarily; however, 52 participants (12%) reported feeling made or pressured to take a test.

One reason given for this was mandatory screening for employment in the private healthcare sector. Nine in ten (91%) participants were currently on antiretroviral treatment; this was similar by gender and ethnicity, and to the overall population accessing HIV care in the UK.

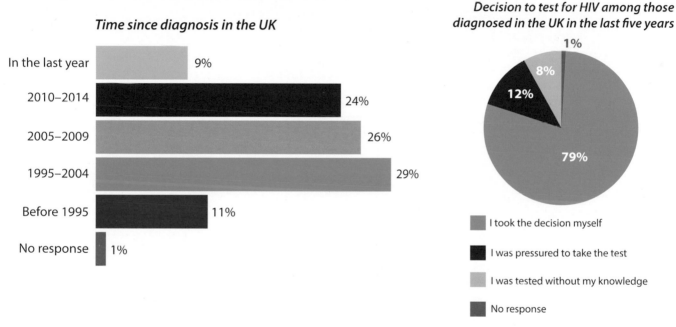

Time since diagnosis in the UK

- In the last year — 9%
- 2010–2014 — 24%
- 2005–2009 — 26%
- 1995–2004 — 29%
- Before 1995 — 11%
- No response — 1%

Decision to test for HIV among those diagnosed in the UK in the last five years

- 79%
- 12%
- 8%
- 1%

- I took the decision myself
- I was pressured to take the test
- I was tested without my knowledge
- No response

Workplace

Almost half (47%) of the 1,059 participants currently working reported that someone in their workplace was aware of their HIV status, while two thirds (63%) felt supported upon telling a co-worker. However, in the last year, 190 (12%) out of all 1,576 participants had decided not to apply for, or turned down, employment or a promotion due to their status.

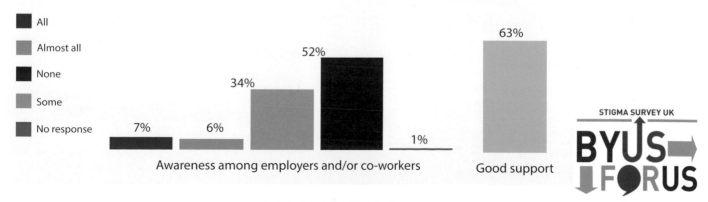

- All
- Almost all
- None
- Some
- No response

7%   6%   34%   52%   1%

Awareness among employers and/or co-workers

63%

Good support

STIGMA SURVEY UK

BYUS FORUS

Experiences of stigma and discrimination

Felt and experienced stigma are affected by many factors, including gender, sexuality, ethnicity and socioeconomic position, along with HIV status. The survey attempted to examine these "layers" of stigma and measure to what extent instances of worry, avoidance and discrimination could be attributed to participants' HIV status.

A significant proportion had worried about being stigmatised, had avoided encounters or had experienced discriminatory treatment in the last 12 months. Many felt this was mainly due to their HIV status (rather than other factors).

Although most participants felt well supported by their partners, relationships provided one of the most common sources of worry in the last year. A third of all participants feared being rejected by a sexual partner (35%) and had avoided sexual encounters (33%) in the last 12 months due to their status.

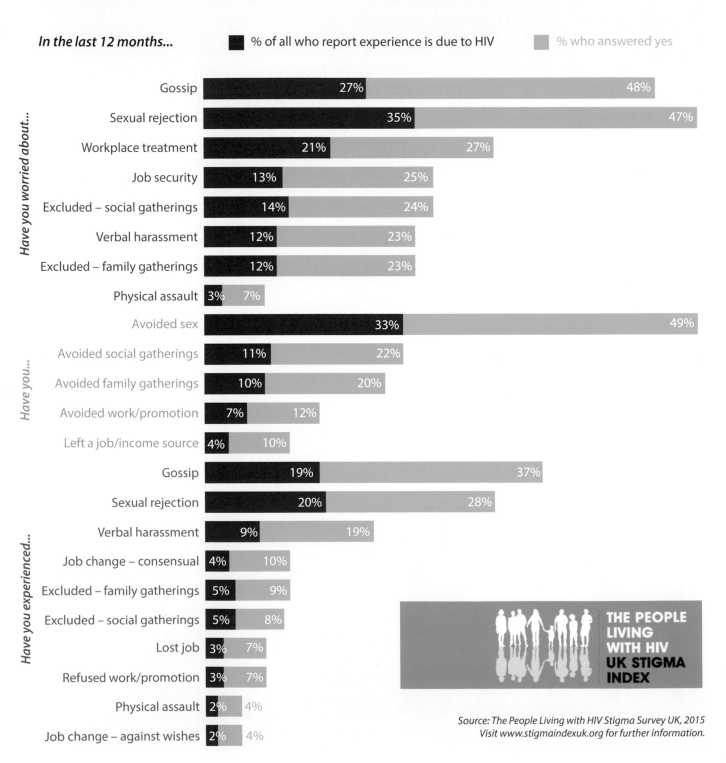

In the last 12 months... ■ % of all who report experience is due to HIV ■ % who answered yes

Have you worried about...

- Gossip — 27% / 48%
- Sexual rejection — 35% / 47%
- Workplace treatment — 21% / 27%
- Job security — 13% / 25%
- Excluded – social gatherings — 14% / 24%
- Verbal harassment — 12% / 23%
- Excluded – family gatherings — 12% / 23%
- Physical assault — 3% / 7%

Have you...

- Avoided sex — 33% / 49%
- Avoided social gatherings — 11% / 22%
- Avoided family gatherings — 10% / 20%
- Avoided work/promotion — 7% / 12%
- Left a job/income source — 4% / 10%

Have you experienced...

- Gossip — 19% / 37%
- Sexual rejection — 20% / 28%
- Verbal harassment — 9% / 19%
- Job change – consensual — 4% / 10%
- Excluded – family gatherings — 5% / 9%
- Excluded – social gatherings — 5% / 8%
- Lost job — 3% / 7%
- Refused work/promotion — 3% / 7%
- Physical assault — 2% / 4%
- Job change – against wishes — 2% / 4%

THE PEOPLE LIVING WITH HIV UK STIGMA INDEX

Source: The People Living with HIV Stigma Survey UK, 2015
Visit www.stigmaindexuk.org for further information.

If my own brother thought he could catch HIV from my towel, imagine what my patients face

He blanched, and took a small step back. Could he catch it from our cups being washed together in the sink? And what about if he touched my towel?

The 'it', of course, was HIV.

I had sustained a needlestick injury. I was almost certain that the test would show I was OK, but we hadn't known the patient had HIV till later, and the one per cent doubt was nagging at me. Telling my parents would not have helped, but I'd wanted to talk things over with my brother.

People's health beliefs are a constant source of wonder. Personal favourites include the young man who assured me you could cure heart attacks by self-performing CPR and the parents who thought grommets meant their child could breathe through his ears. But even so, HIV from towels?

I began to feel guilty at not having taught Pete about HIV myself. Sex education from your sister is not a winning prospect (and one he'd probably have clambered out of windows to avoid) but our secular comp did not do it well.

The biology was taught in mixed-sex classes, with a video so fuzzy that every class ran bets on which figure was female. We never did quite get round to contraception and I may have been off when they did STIs. We were both (just) school-aged in the 90s, though, when the anti-stigma campaigns were in full force and 'My Mummy has AIDS' was a memorable class story. Surely something had to have stuck?

Retrospective education proved of little use; Pete refused to share rooms or meals for the remainder of my visit home and I found him bleaching the cutlery I'd used.

If my graduate brother refused to sit in the same room as me, then what about people going home to tell their partners? My brother was unlikely to erupt into violence: many of my patients have partners who will.

Abroad, I worked with one antenatal service that didn't contact partners after positive tests - the risk of the woman being murdered was too high. Several of my patients assured me that friends and family "would kill them" if they knew their diagnosis. Till now, I'd assumed that was pure hyperbole.

My medic friends were appalled and supportive (mainly offering spoof letters informing Pete that HIV was spread by air). I found myself not telling my other friends, though, afraid of discovering they'd distance themselves, too.

In the end the test was negative, but I still feel grateful to have had that scare. My relationship with Pete may never quite recover but I certainly learned a lot about stigma, and the dangers of assuming people's families will cope when faced with a stigmatised and scary diagnosis.

Tessa Findlay is a junior doctor. She writes under a pseudonym.

24 November 2014

⇨ The above information is reprinted with kind permission from the BMA. Please visit www.bma.org.uk for further information.

© BMA 2017

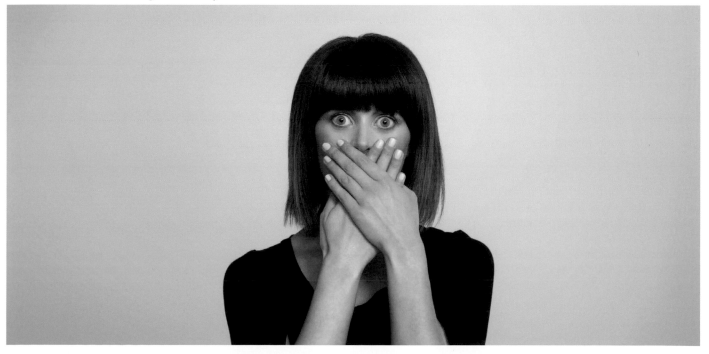

World AIDS Day: after 30 years, the myths and stigma remain - but things can change

By Shaun Griffin

We've come a long way in treating HIV/AIDS in 30 years, but we have a long way to go to fight stigma, writes Shaun Griffin of the Terrence Higgins Trust.

A recognised health issue for the last 30 years, there have been enormous strides taken in HIV treatment since the 1980s. Mostly driven by the increasing range of effective antiretroviral therapies (ART), which lower the amount of HIV in your blood to 'undetectable' levels. As a result there is almost no risk of HIV being passed on.

It is because of ART that HIV is now an entirely manageable health condition. 'Undetectable' women have a very low risk of passing on HIV to their babies. Newborns at risk are given their own short course of the treatment to further reduce their risk of developing HIV, and they undergo a series of tests during the first 18 months of life.

The success of ART led to exploring it as a prevention method (or PrEP) – could using HIV therapy before sex reduce risk of HIV transmission? In February this year, the UK-based PROUD study reported that PrEP reduced the risk of HIV infection by 86 per cent for gay and other men who have sex with men (MSM), when delivered in sexual health clinics in England. PrEP is a game-changer and it is desperately needed in the UK as part of our strategy to defeat HIV.

Last week, French Minister of Health, Marisol Touraine, announced that PrEP will be made accessible throughout the country from 2016 with public funding. The results of two studies – PROUD UK, and Ipergay in France, were considered when making the decision, and used as proof to demonstrate the effectiveness of PrEP as a vital HIV prevention tool.

This is such a huge step forward for European HIV prevention, but a disappointing indicator of where our own government is at. It says a lot that a UK study has, in part, swung the decision for French access, and we are still begging for it here at home.

Though we have achieved great changes in HIV treatment and potential prevention, harder to advance it seems are attitudes to, and public understanding of, HIV. A recent Terrence Higgins Trust snapshot poll, revealed that 90 per cent of people who are living with HIV in Britain think that the public cannot differentiate between HIV and AIDS. It coincides with the #StopStigma effort that the charity is engaging in today, for World AIDS Day.

Also released today, People Living with HIV Stigma Index 2015 survey – the global study of the impact of stigma – found that stigma had prevented 15 per cent of people surveyed from accessing their GP in the last year, and 66 per cent had avoided dental care. 14 per cent had received negative comments from healthcare workers. Whilst most people's GPs were aware of their status, only half felt in control of that disclosure, and the scores were far lower for dental practices.

Those that Terrence Higgins Trust polled were asked for words, unprompted, that they had heard used to describe their health condition. "AIDS", "diseased", "unclean", and "riddled" were among the top four cited. Just a couple of months ago broadcast journalist Kay Burley referred to Dean Street sexual health service as an "AIDS clinic", and was unapologetic.

HIV and AIDS are not the same thing. AIDS is unlikely to develop in people who have been treated in the early stages of HIV infection.

And what of the vile comments during this year's election campaign from Nigel Farrage? He said that immigrants with HIV should not be able to use the UK healthcare system and conjured up 'statistics' in an attempt to defend an unjustifiable point. His claim is completely without evidence and not based on any fact at all. Outrageous.

The respondents to our poll chose an up to date 21st-century public information campaign, and universal testing – making HIV testing the norm in NHS settings, as two important efforts to stop stigma. The latter is already used successfully at St Thomas' Hospital London – one of only two in the entire country who test for HIV as standard in A&E departments.

At Terrence Higgins Trust, we would add a third item to the list – Sex and Relationships Education (SRE). Stigma is manifest in behaviours and attitudes. If we want to achieve comprehensive behaviour change, we need to begin as young as possible. Young people should be given clear and detailed information about the risks of HIV, but also be informed on how living with HIV in the UK has changed, and that it is now an entirely manageable health condition.

For today we can achieve something simple. Change your Facebook or Twitter profile with this and #StopStigma or tweet a picture of you wearing your red ribbon with the same. Let's stand together, today, of all days and #StopStigma.

Shaun Griffin is the Executive Director of External Affairs for the HIV/Aids charity the Terrence Higgins Trust.

December 2015

⇨ The above information is reprinted with kind permission from *The Independent*. Please visit www.independent.co.uk for further information.

© independent.co.uk 2017

Prince Harry's live HIV test creates new demand for home testing kits

Back in July, at the Burrell Street Centre, when Prince Harry took an HIV test live on Facebook, the live streamed event was watched by over two million people. The royal took the test to show how easy it is to be tested. Since then, the demand for at-home HIV test kits has risen 500%.

Campaigners have praised Prince Harry's actions because they've helped not only raise awareness about HIV but helped to do away with the stigmas surrounding the virus. He has been compared by many to his late mother, Diana, Princess of Wales. Out of the 110,000 of those living with HIV, 17% don't know they have the illness.

Prince Harry is very familiar with HIV and AIDS. He's spent time in Africa with Sentebale, the charity he co-founded in Lesotho. A source close to the Prince said: "He has learned a lot about HIV over the last ten years working in Lesotho." They added that Harry is very committed to sticking with this work.

The clinical lead for sexual health at the Burrell Street Centre, Dr Anatole Menon-Johansson, said of the impact Prince Harry's live test has had on not only their clinic but those coming in to be tested: "Prince Harry's visit had a hugely positive impact. Not only have we had more people asking for the test but we've had less resistance to it. One private provider of home testing kits saw a five-fold increase in online orders."

Harry didn't initially intend on taking an HIV test live for all the world to see: "Harry initially came to us to discuss his African charity

Sentebale, which helps the victims of Lesotho's HIV/AIDS epidemic."

He spoke of the Prince's courage to be tested but to also broadcast it live: "Then we started telling him all about one-minute test, and he agreed to do it. It was a brave move, even to be tested, but to then broadcast it on Facebook Live was truly groundbreaking.

"If a Prince can take the test, why not you? Testing is quick, easy and puts you in control."

Ian Green, Chief Executive of Terrence Higgins Trust, said: "It did remind me of his late mother, Princess Diana. She hugged people with AIDS, shook their hands and broke down barriers. We need more people in the limelight like Harry to start these conversations."

He continued by explaining how things haven't changed much in 30 plus years where the illness is concerned and the attitudes of people. Despite all the medical advances, those infected in the UK is at an all-time high, with many not knowing they are.

"Myths, fear and stigma continue to perpetuate the epidemic in the UK.

"People still avoid getting tested for fear of the result, or simply because they don't think HIV is an issue anymore – this causes alarming rates of late diagnosis and means one in six people with HIV don't know they have it.

"Stigma and complacency risk undoing decades of progress."

When Prince Harry took the test: "It showed the world that an HIV test is nothing to be feared or ashamed of," said Dr Anatole Menon-Johansson. He called the Prince's actions a "turning point."

He said, "If you get a positive result, you can get onto treatment that enables you to live a normal healthy life, and prevents you from passing on the virus."

Prince Harry will mark World AIDS Day on 1 December while in Barbados. He will lead a discussion about HIV with the youth there. Earlier this month, Elton John helped Harry campaign about HIV. The singer/songwriter also had high praise for the royal. Elton John said, "People love him because he has his mother's ability to communicate so brilliantly on a very, very humble level.

"[Diana] had that ability to walk into a room and make people feel very at ease and he does that too.

"[Harry's] great because he appeals to young people. I'm a little old, so I can't get through to the people that he can get to.

"We need more people like that to get through to young people because infections among young people are growing, not falling."

29 November 2016

⇨ The above information is reprinted with kind permission from Royal Central. Please visit www.royalcentral.co.uk for further information.

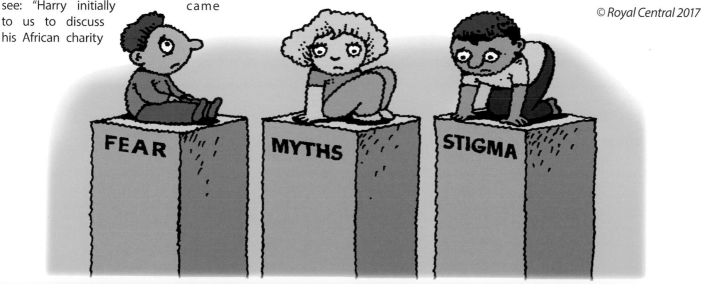

Social care must shed HIV myths to support first ageing generation

The social care sector needs education in the realities of HIV to support the first generation to grow older with the condition, writes Alice Booth.

Care homes and HIV

These aren't generally terms one expects to hear in the same sentence; but in the not-too-distant future, they will be.

Thanks to medical advances, people with HIV are living longer than ever before. This is extremely positive news – but it also means we are entering uncharted territory. The fastest growing group of people in the UK living with HIV is the over-50s, representing one third of those affected.

Within the next two decades, we will have an acute problem in terms of how we support this new and fast-growing population and I'm not sure the social care sector is ready.

Perfect storm

A perfect storm is brewing. We've got more and more people facing old age while living with HIV, a highly stigmatised and misunderstood condition, while we have exactly zero experience of HIV in older age.

At the same time, we have a social care sector that's already busting at the seams. There is chronic loneliness and poverty among the ageing HIV population, as was been revealed in a recent Terrence Higgins Trust report, *Uncharted Territory*. We could see a real crisis within the next few years, as more of those diagnosed at the start of the epidemic enter their 70s, 80s and 90s.

It's a particular issue where I work in Brighton, where we have the second highest HIV prevalence outside London. I've worked in HIV for four years, and recently I've been co-ordinating the Terrence Higgins Trust's Health, Wealth and Happiness Project for the over-50s.

Isolation and anxiety

Many of my clients are older gay men, who were diagnosed in the 1980s and 1990s, before HIV treatment was available and life expectancy was only a few years. Many of these clients don't have family support, and many have become isolated due to fear of social rejection.

I hear a lot of anxiety from clients about having to go back into the closet if they go into a care home, and then on top of that having to disclose their HIV status in an environment where it might be shared, and where they may be ostracised from their peers. Some worry they'd need to hide their medication from home carers for fear of their reaction.

In 2017, this shouldn't be an issue. But it is.

On top of this, many cashed in their pensions when they were told they were facing a death sentence. Here they are today and 88% haven't made any financial plans concerning their future care.

My role is to address the complex needs of people ageing with HIV and help them to live well, while facing the uncertainty of what lies ahead. We hold wellbeing days, group support sessions and workshops covering everything from how to order shopping online, to financial arrangements like wills and pensions.

HIV myths

A key part of my role is delivering training on HIV awareness within care homes and other social care providers. I've actually been pleasantly surprised by how receptive they've been towards the training – but during the sessions, you nearly always hear staff repeat the same myths around HIV that you still hear from the general public. These myths were widespread in the 1980s and are still deeply entrenched today.

For example, we're often asked, "do I need to wear two pairs of gloves while giving personal care if my client has HIV?", or "do I need to disclose the client's HIV status to all staff working in the care home?".

My answers are simple: no, and no.

There is no reason to treat someone living with HIV any differently, other than to support them to take their medication and to be mindful of the potential for stigma and discrimination.

You cannot transmit HIV from skin-to-skin contact or from saliva. The virus does not survive long outside the body so you cannot get HIV from towels, toilet seats or any other household item.

No risk of transmission

But most importantly (and this is where things have changed far more swiftly than public awareness) people who are on effective HIV treatment cannot pass on the virus at all. This is because current HIV treatment works by reducing the amount of the virus to undetectable (and therefore uninfectious) levels. If more people knew this, the stigma would surely decrease.

Older people living with HIV aren't a tricky or problematic group. Usually, getting it right is just common sense. It's a case of respecting their confidentiality, ensuring you have an up-to-date understanding of HIV, and supporting them to access local resources and networks, like the Health, Wealth and Happiness Project.

But most importantly I think it's about remembering that your client is part of the first generation facing old age with HIV. We know this is coming and those working in social care are getting more and more likely to encounter someone with these needs.

As social care professionals, as charities and as members of society, we must be thinking ahead – and we must stand with this new community as they face the path untrodden.

Alice Booth is coordinator of the Health, Wealth and Happiness project run by the Terrence Higgins Trust in Brighton.

2 February 2017

⇨ The above information is reprinted with kind permission from Community Care. Please visit www.communitycare.co.uk.

London should have an AIDS memorial – and the Assembly just voted to support it

The UK has no national memorial to victims of the epidemic.

By Sian Berry

I was very happy to see the London Assembly unanimously back the idea of a national HIV/AIDS memorial in London this week.

The idea for a national memorial to recognise those who died from HIV and AIDS was revived by Gay Men Fighting AIDS (GMFA) and they have been leading the campaign to make this memorial a reality.

The concept has been talked about for years, and meanwhile many other cities worldwide have finished and opened similar memorials, most recently New York.

Now GMFA, in conjunction with the UK HIV sector, have revived the campaign and obtained thousands of signatories for a petition. I was proud to propose a motion to the London Assembly last month.

To get this passed unanimously is a strong statement of political support, which will add to the growing momentum behind this idea.

The long list of supporters collected by GMFA so far stretches from clinicians who worked through the epidemic, activist groups like Act Up and UK Black Pride, charities including the British HIV Association and The Haemophilia Society, and the mayor's own Night Tsar, Amy Lamé.

We do need this in London. Our city was hardest hit by the epidemic in the UK, not just among the LGBT community but among people with haemophilia, new African communities, prisoners and injecting drug users.

The effects of that terrible epidemic are still keenly felt today by those who lost loved ones to HIV and AIDS, as well as many people still living with this diagnosis.

London is also home to the pioneering 56 Dean St Clinic which I visited last year

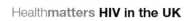

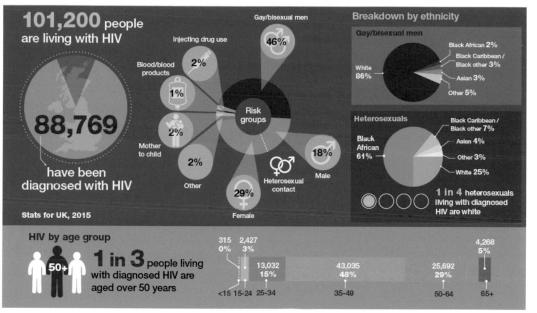

and which has demonstrated enormous progress in preventing new infections in recent months.

It is wonderful that people in the UK newly diagnosed with HIV can presume a normal life expectancy. But access to life-prolonging medication is not yet universal. London's global reach means we have strong ties to communities still disproportionately suffering from AIDS and HIV.

But the memorial is not just about the people lost to a terrible disease. The AIDS epidemic profoundly challenged a lot of prejudices in our society and continues to do so more than 30 years later. This work must continue, and the memorial would serve a valuable purpose in recognising the importance of these events and continuing to educate people and break down stigma.

Yesterday I was very touched to see Assembly Members from across the political spectrum add their support and give moving speeches of their personal experiences. AIDS has affected so many people and testimonials from Assembly Members who were former healthcare workers

and those who lost friends and former partners, showed.

The mayor recently expressed support for the petition and wished the campaign every success. He promised to stay involved as the project develops. It is my hope that the backing from the mayor and the London Assembly helps build momentum to take the campaign to the next phase in encouraging potential backers and the Government to provide funding.

I first supported a memorial during the election campaign last year and it was a shock then to find out that the UK didn't already have a national memorial. I hope we're now one step closer to that.

Sian Berry is a Green member of the London Assembly.

10 February 2017

⇨ The above information is reprinted with kind permission from Left Foot Forward. Please visit www.leftfootforward.org for further information.

Treating HIV

There is no cure for HIV, but there are treatments to enable most people with the virus to live a long and healthy life.

Emergency HIV drugs

If you think you have been exposed to the virus within the last 72 hours (three days), anti-HIV medication may stop you becoming infected.

For it to be effective, the medication, called post-exposure prophylaxis or PEP, must be started within 72 hours of coming into contact with the virus. It is only recommended following higher risk exposure, particularly where the sexual partner is known to be positive.

The quicker PEP is started the better, ideally within hours of coming into contact with HIV. The longer the wait, the less chance of it being effective.

PEP has been misleadingly popularised as a 'morning-after pill' for HIV – a reference to the emergency pill women can take to prevent getting pregnant after having unprotected sex.

But the description is not accurate. PEP is a month-long treatment, which may have serious side effects and is not guaranteed to work. The treatment involves taking the same drugs prescribed to people who have tested positive for HIV.

You should be able to get PEP from:

⇨ sexual health clinics, or genitourinary medicine (GUM) clinics

⇨ hospitals – usually accident and emergency (A&E) departments.

If you already have HIV, try your HIV clinic if the PEP is for someone you've had sex with.

If you test positive

If you are diagnosed with HIV, you will have regular blood tests to monitor the progress of the HIV infection before starting treatment.

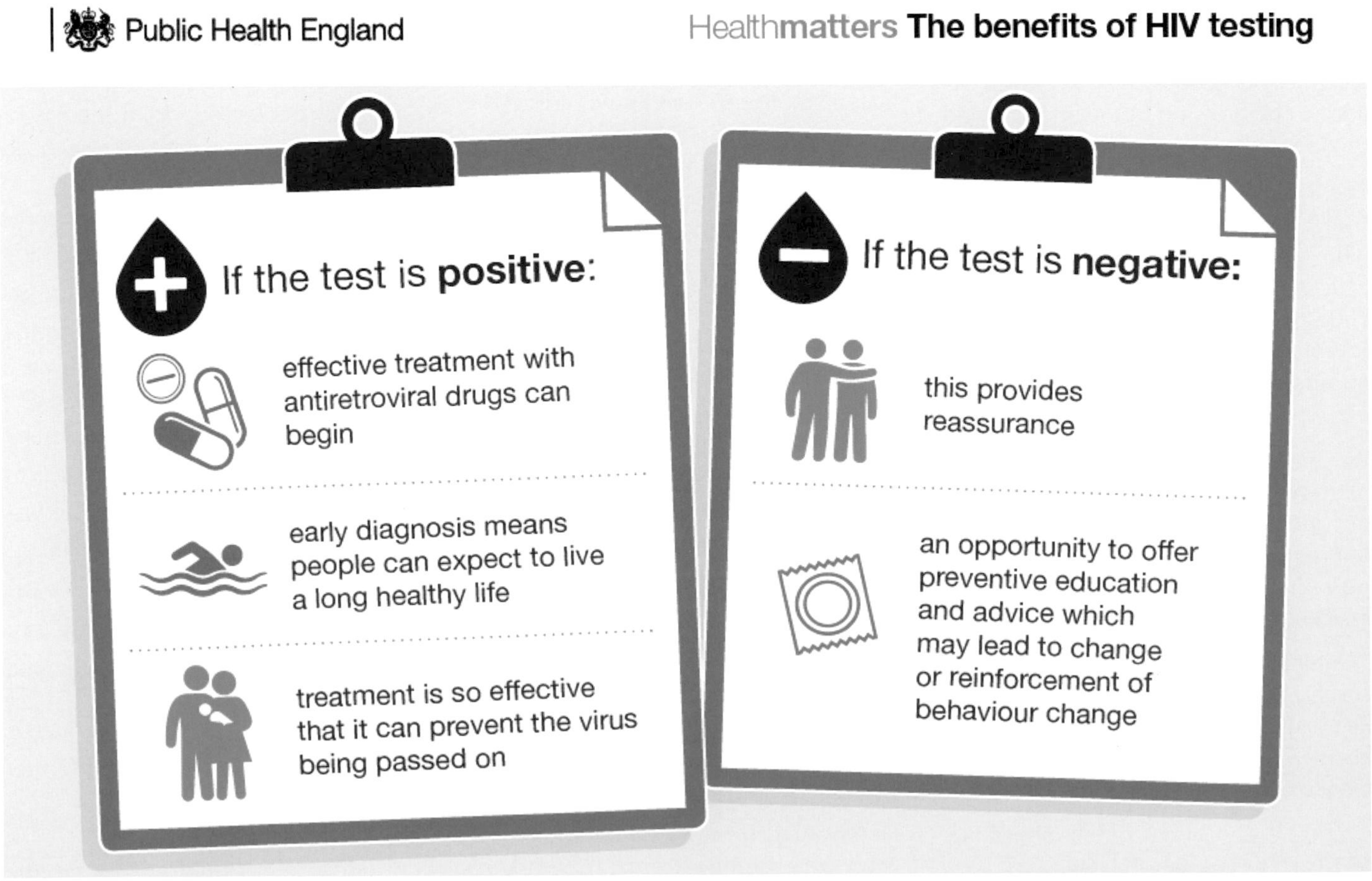

Public Health England

Healthmatters **The benefits of HIV testing**

If the test is **positive:**

- effective treatment with antiretroviral drugs can begin
- early diagnosis means people can expect to live a long healthy life
- treatment is so effective that it can prevent the virus being passed on

If the test is **negative:**

- this provides reassurance
- an opportunity to offer preventive education and advice which may lead to change or reinforcement of behaviour change

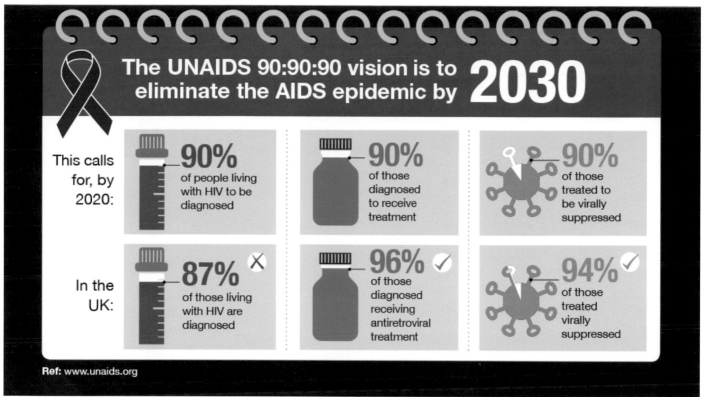

The UNAIDS 90:90:90 vision is to eliminate the AIDS epidemic by 2030

This calls for, by 2020:
- **90%** of people living with HIV to be diagnosed
- **90%** of those diagnosed to receive treatment
- **90%** of those treated to be virally suppressed

In the UK:
- **87%** of those living with HIV are diagnosed ✗
- **96%** of those diagnosed receiving antiretroviral treatment ✓
- **94%** of those treated virally suppressed ✓

Ref: www.unaids.org

This involves monitoring the amount of virus in your blood (viral blood test) and the effect HIV is having on your immune system. This is determined by measuring your levels of CD4+ve lymphocyte cells in your blood. These cells are important for fighting infection.

Treatment is usually recommended to begin when your CD4 cell count falls towards 350 or below, whether or not you have any symptoms. In some people with other medical conditions, treatment may be started at higher CD4 cell counts. When to start treatment should be discussed with your doctor.

The aim of the treatment is to reduce the level of HIV in the blood, allow the immune system to repair itself and prevent any HIV-related illnesses.

If you are on HIV treatment, the level of the virus in your blood is generally very low and it is unlikely that you will pass HIV on to someone else.

If you have another condition

If you have also been diagnosed with hepatitis B or hepatitis C, it is recommended that you start treatment when your CD4 count falls below 500.

Treatment is recommended to begin at any CD4 count if you are on radiotherapy or chemotherapy that will suppress your immune system, or if you have been diagnosed with certain other illnesses, including:

⇨ tuberculosis

⇨ HIV-related nephropathy (kidney disease)

⇨ HIV-related neurocognitive (brain) illnesses.

Antiretroviral drugs

HIV is treated with antiretrovirals (ARVs), these work by stopping the virus replicating in the body, allowing the immune system to repair itself and preventing further damage.

A combination of ARVs is used because HIV can quickly adapt and become resistant to one single ARV.

Patients tend to take three or more types of ARV medication. This is known as combination therapy or antiretroviral therapy (ART).

Some antiretroviral drugs have been combined into one pill, known as a 'fixed dose combination'. This means that the most common treatments for people just diagnosed with HIV

involve taking just one or two pills a day.

Different combinations of ARVs work for different people so the medicine you take will be individual to you.

Once HIV treatment is started, you will probably need to take the medication for the rest of your life. For the treatment to be continuously effective, it will need to be taken regularly every day. Not taking ARVs regularly may cause the treatment to fail.

Many of the medicines used to treat HIV can interact with other medications prescribed by your GP or bought over-the-counter. These include herbal remedies such as St John's Wort, as well as recreational drugs.

Always check with your HIV clinic staff or your GP before taking any other medicines.

Pregnancy

ARV treatment is available to prevent a pregnant woman from passing HIV to her child.

Without treatment, there is a one in four chance your baby will become infected with HIV. With treatment, the risk is less than one in 100.

Advances in treatment mean there is no increased risk of passing the virus to your baby with a normal delivery. However, for some women, a caesarean section may still be recommended.

If you have HIV, do not breastfeed your baby because the virus can be transmitted through breast milk.

If you or your partner has HIV, speak to an HIV doctor as there are options for safely conceiving a child without putting either of you at risk of infection.

Missing a dose

HIV treatment only works if you take your pills regularly every day. Missing even a few doses will increase the risk of your treatment not working.

You will need to develop a daily routine to fit your treatment plan around your lifestyle.

Side effects

HIV treatment can have side effects. If you get serious side effects (which is uncommon) you may need to try a different combination of ARVs.

Common side effects include:

⇨ nausea

⇨ diarrhoea

⇨ skin rashes

⇨ sleep difficulties.

People with HIV get treatment at a specialist HIV clinic which is usually part of a sexual health or infectious diseases clinic at your local hospital.

Services, including support organisations, may work together to provide specialist care and emotional support.

8 September 2016

⇨ The above information is reprinted with kind permission from NHS Choices. Please visit www.nhs.uk for further information.

© NHS Choices 2017

'Treat all' to end AIDS

Achieving the global target to end AIDS by 2030 will require rapid and effective implementation of the World Health Organization's (WHO) 'treat all' recommendations, as noted by delegates from countries and partner organizations at the United Nations High-Level Meeting on Ending AIDS. At the end of 2015, more than 17 million people were receiving antiretroviral therapy out of a total 37 million people living with HIV.

Opening the WHO side event *Treat all: from policy to action – what will it take?*, the Director of the WHO HIV Department, Dr Gottfried Hirnschall said, "Over the past ten months, an encouraging number of countries have introduced 'treat all' policies and began implementation, which is a great start," said Dr Hirnschall.

As of June 2016, close to 80 low- and middle-income countries have adopted 'treat all' policies or announced plans to do so within the year. Of these countries, 24 have already started implementation of 'treat all' policies.

At the event, WHO released the full version of the second edition of the *Consolidated guidelines on the use of antiretroviral drugs for treating and preventing HIV infection: recommendations for a public health approach.*

Published in June 2016, the guidelines contain key recommendations to 'treat all' people living with HIV, including children, adolescents, adults, pregnant and breastfeeding women, and people with coinfections. They also include new service delivery recommendations on how to expand coverage of HIV treatment to reach all people living with HIV.

The recommendations aim to improve the quality of HIV treatment and to bring us closer to the universal health coverage ideals of integrated services, community-centred and community-led health care approaches, and shared responsibility for effective programme delivery.

9 June 2016

⇨ The above information is reprinted with kind permission from the World Health Organization. Please visit www.who.int for further information.

⇨ Reprinted from http://www.who.int/hiv/mediacentre/news/arv-2016-launch/en/ [03 May 2017].

© World Health Organization 2017

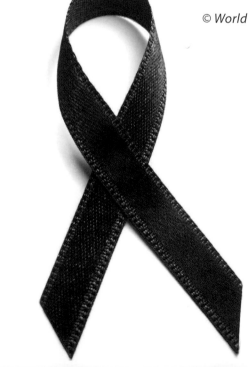

WHO confirms antiretroviral therapy reduces the risk of life-threatening HIV-related infections

Adults and children with HIV who start antiretroviral therapy (ART) as early as possible reduce their risk of developing serious HIV-related infections, according to new findings published in the journal **Clinical Infectious Diseases** *on 15 June 2016.*

Two studies in adults and children, supported by the World Health Organization (WHO) and conducted in collaboration with Columbia University, the London School of Hygiene & Tropical Medicine and McGill University, are the first global systematic and comprehensive analyses of data on HIV-related opportunistic infections over a 20-year period in three global regions: Africa, Asia and Latin America. The two reviews compared the risk of serious HIV-related infections before and after starting ART, then estimated the global number of cases of infection that would have been prevented (using data from 2013), and the costs saved, if ART had been started earlier.

"Opportunistic and other infections are the major cause of death in adults and children with HIV," said Dr Philippa Easterbrook from WHO's Department of HIV. "There have been previous estimates on the impact of ART in reducing deaths and new HIV infections, but not on its impact on each of the serious infections to which people with HIV are vulnerable, especially in low-income settings. Knowing how common these infections are is really important for planning HIV health services in these countries, including procuring drugs and diagnostic tests."

In 126 different studies based on almost half a million adult HIV patients, the most common infections were oral thrush, tuberculosis, shingles and bacterial pneumonia – each of which occurred in more than 5% of adults before ART. There was a major reduction in the risk of development of all infections for those on ART, by 57% to 91%, and this was greatest in the first year of treatment. It was estimated that earlier ART would have prevented at least 900,000 cases of life-threatening infections and saved around US$50 million in 2013.

In the second review – 88 studies based on 55,679 HIV-infected children – bacterial pneumonia and tuberculosis were the most common infections, each occurring in around 25% of children before ART. As with the adult studies, there was a reduction in risk for all infections for those on ART, but this was greatest (by more than 80%) for HIV-related diarrhoea, cerebral toxoplasmosis and tuberculosis, with a smaller impact on bacterial septicaemia and pneumonia. It was estimated that earlier access to ART could have prevented at least 161,000 cases of serious infections in children, with a saving of around US$17 million in 2013.

"Compared to adults, there is always a relative lack of data on HIV-infected children to inform guidelines and practice, and the scale-up of ART in children has been much less successful," said coauthor Dr Marie-Renée B-Lajoie from McGill University. "But our study shows that the effect of ART in reducing HIV-related infections in children is as dramatic as that seen in adults."

Dr Andrea Low, coauthor from ICAP, Columbia University, commented that "the level of effect of ART on serious infections in adults in these low-income settings was even more striking than that observed in high-income countries". However, she also noted that interpretation of regional variation in incidence and the effect of ART is limited, as there were significant gaps in data from some regions, such as Latin America.

Dr Gottfried Hirnschall, Director of WHO's HIV Department, concluded: "We know that ART has a dramatic effect in reducing death rates as well as new HIV infections. These findings demonstrate that ART has the same effect in reducing the risk of serious HIV-relatedl infections in adults and children – thus, further explaining the reduction in death rates. This reinforces the need to continually prioritise the expansion of access to ART. The new WHO guidelines recommend starting ART in all HIV-infected persons as soon as possible, regardless of the stage of infection."

20 June 2016

⇨ The above information is reprinted with kind permission from the World Health Organization. Please visit www.who.int for further information.

⇨ Reprinted from http://www.who.int/hiv/mediacentre/ news/incidence-oi-impact-art-news/en/ [03 May 2017].

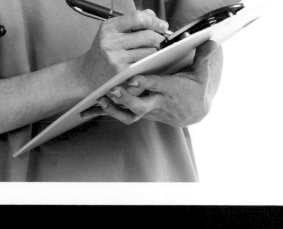

Breaking negative attitudes to women is key to tackling HIV – here's how to do it

An article from **The Conversation.**

THE CONVERSATION

Tanya Abramsky, Research Fellow in Epidemiology, London School of Hygiene & Tropical Medicine

" Women are supposed to be under men's superiority in everything… you cannot respond when he says anything. You only have to do what he says." That's what one young woman told staff at Raising Voices, a Ugandan violence prevention charity, that she used to think before she became a community activist. Sadly, throughout many parts of the world, such views are still common.

These beliefs are also fuelling an epidemic of HIV in women – limiting women's access to education and economic opportunities, condoning men's use of violence against them, and ultimately making it difficult for women to refuse sex or request condom use.

HIV is now the leading cause of death and sickness among women of reproductive age in low- and middle-income countries. In Sub-Saharan Africa, the region most affected by HIV, adolescent and young women bear the heaviest burden – they are twice as likely to become infected as their male peers.

Current approaches to tackling the epidemic just don't seem to be enough. "Right now what we do with HIV is we tell people they should use condoms," explains Lori Heise, research director of STRIVE, an international research consortium led by the London School of Hygiene & Tropical Medicine, "but sometimes people are living in contexts where making the healthy choice is very difficult… because of poverty, because of gender norms and the degree to which women are disadvantaged in society."

Empowering women

These gender norms that promote men's dominance over women are now a growing focus of HIV prevention efforts. So, can we change these norms? And if so, how?

Addressing multiple strands of female disadvantage simultaneously has been shown to be very effective. IMAGE, a programme for rural South African women, combined microfinance – small loans to start businesses or other income-generating activities – with socially empowering group learning sessions which covered topics ranging from gender and cultural beliefs to domestic violence and HIV. It proved a winning combination. Rates of partner violence against women were halved, and younger women became less likely to have unprotected sex and more likely to access HIV testing.

Of course, it's not just women that we need to focus on. A whole series of behaviours that some men equate with 'being a man' – having multiple sexual partners, visiting sex-workers, binge drinking and using violence against their female partners – increase those men's risk of acquiring HIV and passing the infection on to their female partners. Clearly, the best way to challenge such notions of manhood is to target young men and adolescent boys.

Programme H, developed by a Brazilian NGO, is now used in over 22 countries. The programme engages adolescent boys and young men in months of interactive group sessions focused on, among other topics, gender, sexuality, fatherhood, violence and HIV. In its various incarnations, Programme H has succeeded in changing gender attitudes, improving relationships, reducing violence against women and increasing condom use.

It may also have led to a decrease in sexually transmitted diseases, as fewer symptoms have been reported. However, the incidence of HIV has not yet been investigated. Adaptations of Programme H that have proved most successful have used youth-led community campaigns to make sure that peers are receptive to the ideas and behaviours of boys who have been through the programme.

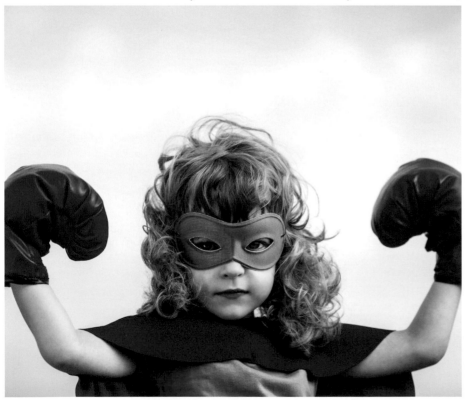

Community effort

The importance of what the wider community thinks and does cannot be understated. This makes a newer approach, community mobilisation, one of the most exciting – albeit challenging – approaches out there. But it is achievable, as demonstrated by two programmes in Uganda – SASA! in urban Kampala, and SHARE in rural Rakai.

Community activists are vital players in this type of intervention – regular men and women from the community trained up alongside local government, cultural leaders, police and healthcare providers, to deliver activities within their own neighbourhoods. Through thousands of activities and encounters – ranging from community meetings and door-to-door discussions to community dramas, informal chats at taxi ranks and consultations with traditional marriage counsellors – the programme takes on a life of its own.

Change doesn't happen overnight, but it can happen impressively quickly. After three years, SASA! halved the rates of physical partner violence against women. Women felt more able to refuse sex, and men became less likely to have multiple concurrent sexual partners. SHARE strikingly reduced both partner violence and rates of new HIV infection among community members.

As great minds converge on Durban, South Africa, this week for the biennial International AIDS conference, there is reason for optimism, but no place for complacency. Urgent questions should be high up the agenda. How can we deliver promising programmes on a larger scale? What opportunities are there to better integrate violence and HIV prevention programming? And how can we ensure norm-changing programmes are adequately funded and taken to scale?

The answers may not come easily, but in the words of a SASA! activist, "What used to be done by our ancestors can be changed." And that change can't come soon enough for the millions of women in this world who are living in the shadow of HIV.

19 July 2016

⇨ The above information is reprinted with kind permission from *The Conversation*. Please visit www.theconversation.com for further information.

In surprise decision, UK government rejects plans to add PrEP to National Health Service

"Today's decision by NHS England... is shameful," said Ian Green, director of the Terrence Higgins Trust.

By Dan Avery

This week activists and medical experts were stunned to hear the British Government has decided to scratch plans to put PrEP on the National Health Service.

It has, instead, approved £2 million for "early-implementer tests" that would provide pre-exposure prophylaxis to 500 men at high risk of HIV infection.

In a statement, NHS England said getting the drug to at-risk communities was not its responsibility, though it was "committed to working with local authorities, Public Health England, the Department of Health and other stakeholders" on the issue.

Activists complain the £2 million allotment is arbitrary, especially when PrEP has already proven effective – both in the UK and abroad.

"NHS England led us to believe for the last two years that they would be willing to commission and fund PrEP as long as it met the appropriate criteria of cost effectiveness," said Yusef Azad of the National AIDS Trust. He blasted today's decision as "another example of our health system refusing to fund prevention effectively" and complained that it's still not clear who's responsibility it is to get PrEP greenlighted.

"Is it the Department of Health, local authorities, the NHS or Public Health England? We need answers, we need access, and we demand both."

"By denying full availability of PrEP we are failing those who are at risk of HIV," said Ian Green, CEO of the Terrence Higgins Trust, a major AIDS organisation in the UK.

"Today's decision by NHS England to depart with due process, and, instead, offer a tokenistic nod to what has the potential to revolutionise HIV prevention in the UK, is shameful."

More than 2,500 men who have sex with men are diagnosed with HIV each year in the UK, a figure that has remained constant over the past ten years.

22 March 2016

⇨ The above information is reprinted with kind permission from New Now Next. Please visit www.newnownext.com for further information.

Norway becomes first country to provide free PrEP

"We are happy that PrEP is now an integrated part of the public health service."

By Cody Gohl

In a powerful show of support for its LGBT community, the Norwegian Government has become the first country in the world to offer PrEP free of charge as part of its National Health Service.

The Pre-exposure Prophylaxis (PrEP) drug Truvada has been proven to reduce the risk of HIV infection by 86 per cent and has been endorsed by the World Health Organization and the Centers for Disease Control and Prevention.

The drug is available in a number of countries, including the United States, Canada, France, South Africa and, now, Norway.

Minister for Health and Social Care Bent Høie made the announcement earlier this week, stating that the drug would not only be available in the country, but that it would also be provided to at-risk users at no expense.

The landmark move came as the result of two years of tireless lobbying by HIV Norway in conjunction with the Institute of Public Health and the Health Directorate.

"PrEP will contribute to reducing the rate of new infections in the gay community, as gay men are facing a risk of infection much higher than the general population," stated Leif-Ove Hansen, the president of HIV Norway.

"Condom use is on the decline," he continued, "and we are happy that PrEP now is an integrated part of the public health service."

The bold decision has been met with great enthusiasm from HIV charities around the world, many of whom are still advocating for PrEP to become available in their countries.

Ian Green, Chief Executive of Terrence Higgins Trust in the UK, said: "Norway's decision to provide PrEP is another great step forward for HIV prevention in Europe. PrEP is a game changer and, when used alongside condoms, regular testing and effective treatment, it can help end the HIV epidemic for good."

"[Governments] must stop with their delays and confusion," he concluded, "and make PrEP immediately available to those at risk of HIV."

20 October 2016

⇨ The above information is reprinted with kind permission from New Now Next. Please visit www.newnownext.com for further information.

A new HIV vaccine could be the "final nail in the coffin" for the disease

"It would significantly decrease the burden of HIV."

By Sophie Gallagher

A new vaccine being tested in South Africa could be the "nail in the coffin" of HIV as it helps to protect people against contracting the disease.

The disease, which attacks the autoimmune system, affects an estimated 103,700 people in the UK alone, according to the NHS.

But a new vaccine, HVTN 702, could significantly decrease the number of people contracting HIV around the world, as it is able to help prevent infection.

Anthony Fauci, director of the US Government's National Institute of Allergy and Infectious Disease: "If deployed alongside our current armoury of proven HIV prevention tools, a safe and effective vaccine could be the final nail in the coffin for HIV."

Scientists in Johannesburg are basing the current trial on research from a similar 2009 study done in Thailand that showed HVTN 702 was 31.2% effective at preventing HIV infection over 3.5 years.

The team aim to enrol 5,400 sexually active men and women, aged 18–35, and give them five injections (either vaccine or placebo) in the largest ever HIV clinical trial to take place in the country.

Results are expected to be published in 2020, and Fauci says that even moderate success would be something to celebrate.

"Even a moderately effective vaccine would significantly decrease the burden of HIV disease over time in countries and populations with high rates of HIV infection, such as South Africa."

28 November 2016

⇨ The above information is reprinted with kind permission from The Huffington Post UK. Please visit www.huffingtonpost.co.uk for further information.

The latest breakthroughs in AIDS and HIV research in 2016

This year has seen promising steps towards a cure for HIV and AIDS, but we're not there yet.

By Martha Henriques

Here are five of the biggest research breakthroughs relating to HIV and AIDS.

1. Antiretroviral therapies confirmed to be highly effective

A pair of studies from the World Health Organization found that antiretroviral therapies are effective at reducing HIV infections and deaths from AIDS.

At the end of 2015 almost half of the estimated 37 million people living with HIV were receiving antiretroviral therapy.

Antiretroviral therapies stop the proliferation of HIV in the body to reduce the viral load. This greatly reduces the risk of transmitting the virus to more people. If both sexual partners are receiving antiretroviral therapy then the likelihood of transmission can be reduced by up to 96 per cent.

It's thought that antiretroviral therapy has saved nearly eight million lives so far.

2. Antibody treatment proves effective HIV treatment for those who resist antiretroviral therapy

A Phase III clinical trial has found that people who do not respond to antiretroviral therapy can be treated with monoclonal antibodies.

Antiretroviral therapy has several side effects, such as anaemia, nausea and diarrhoea. Some patients do not respond to these therapies at all. Research has shown that monoclonal antibodies could soon be an alternative treatment option for people diagnosed with HIV.

The treatment has yet to be approved by the Food and Drug Administration in the US.

3. Antibody therapy could boost immune system to help patients off antiretrovirals

Antibody therapies could also help as an additional treatment to antiretrovirals.

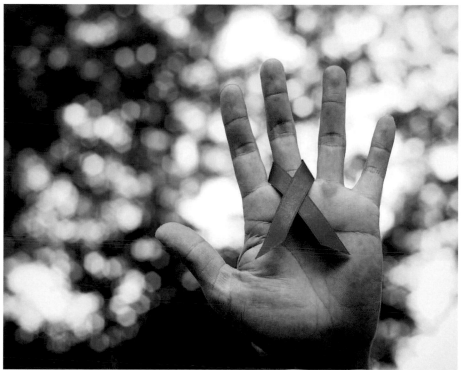

Monkeys that had the simian equivalent of HIV – SIV – had their viral load reduced to undetectable levels after receiving the antibody anti-alpha4/beta7 after receiving antiretroviral therapy.

The paper, published in the journal *Science*, found that after receiving the antibody once a fortnight for 32 weeks, high levels of SIV did not return in the monkeys when antiretroviral therapy was stopped.

A pilot clinical trial of the therapy in humans is now underway.

4. Gene-editing technology used for HIV research

The use of precise gene-editing technology in HIV research could hasten the search for a cure for HIV and Aids. Researchers at the University of California San Francisco used CRISPR-Cas9 technology to investigate human immune cells' resistance to HIV.

They found that mutations in two genes – CXCR4 and CCR5 – offered some protection to HIV. This research will now form the basis for further studies into whether this can be converted into an effective treatment.

5. Crucial HIV protein structure seen up close

The protein that allows HIV to recognise and infect human immune cells was identified in high resolution for the first time. In a study published in the journal *Science*, researchers modelled the protein in its natural form.

This could help medical researchers identify antibodies that could target the protein to stop the virus before it can infiltrate the immune system.

30 November 2016

⇨ The above information is reprinted with kind permission from the *International Business Times*. Please visit www.ibtimes.co.uk for further information.

Every tenth child in South Africa has innate AIDS defence

A study found that one in ten children have a "monkey-like" immune system that stops them developing AIDS.

By Dragana Todorovic

Scientists have analysed the blood of 170 children from South Africa with HIV who have never had treatment nor developed AIDS. The tests showed that the respondents had tens of thousands of human immunodeficiency viruses in every millilitre of their blood. Normally this would push their immune system over the limit of endurance as the body would be trying to fight the infection, but that was not happening. The fact that the immune system had not attacked the virus, saved it.

According to the study published in the journal *Science Translational Medicine*, every one in ten children has an immune system that keeps them from developing AIDS.

The study found that the immune system in these children remained inactive, similar to monkeys, which prevented it from being wiped out.

An untreated HIV infection is fatal in 60 per cent of children within two and a half years, but it is interesting that an identical infection in monkeys is not fatal. This finding could lead to a new immune therapy for HIV infection.

Professor Philip Goulder, one of the researchers from the University of Oxford, explained to the BBC that the immune system of these children ignores the virus for as long as possible. Warfare against the virus in most cases is absolutely the wrong thing, the professor said.

HIV kills white blood cells, the immune system's fighters. And when the body's defences go into overdrive, even more of these cells are killed. According to Goulder, one of the things to come out of this new study is that the disease is not so much to do with HIV, but to the immune response to it.

The way that ten percent of children cope with the virus has striking similarities to the way more than 40 non-human primate species cope with simian immunodeficiency virus or SIV.

They have had tens of thousands of years to develop a way to fight the infection. This defence against AIDS is almost unique to children.

In adult humans, the immune system tends to go all out in an effort to finish the virus, which in most cases ends in failure. Children have relatively tolerant immune systems, which become more aggressive in adulthood – measles, for example, is far more severe in adults due to the way their immune system responds. This does not mean that as they get older these kids will develop AIDS. Some will, but some will not get AIDS.

Dr Ann Chahroudi and Dr Guido Silvestri, from Emory University in the United States, explained that the study may have found the very earliest signs of coevolution of HIV in humans, the BBC reports.

They added that it is not known whether it would be clinically safe for these newly identified HIV infected paediatric non-progressors to remain off-therapy.

"This assessment is further complicated by the fact that prevention of HIV transmission to sexual partners becomes relevant in adolescence," they added in a commentary.

Prof. Goulder said that he believes these findings in children could ultimately help rebalance the immune system in all HIV patients.

8 October 2016

⇨ The above information is reprinted with kind permission from Newswire. Please visit www.newswire.net for further information.

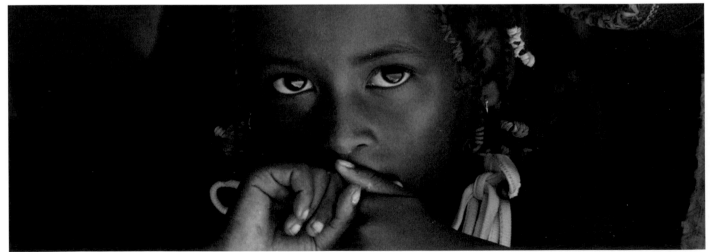

Helping HIV patients experience happiness could be key to boosting their physical health

Participants were asked to recognise a positive event each day.

By Rachel Moss

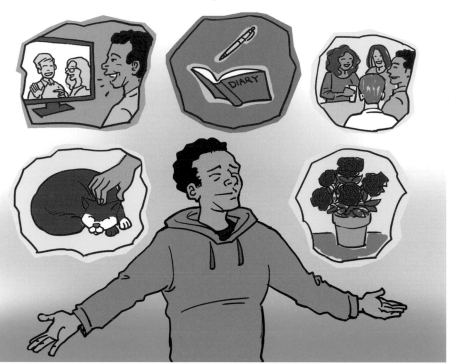

Helping people with HIV to feel emotionally happy could help to improve their physical symptoms, new research suggests.

A study found that when individuals recently diagnosed with HIV were coached to practise skills to help them experience positive emotions, the result was less HIV in their blood and lower antidepressant use.

Coaching included focusing on positive events, through popular diaries called gratitude journals.

The researchers, from Northwestern Medicine, said the findings could pave the way for new intervention treatments for people in the initial stages of adjustment to any serious chronic illness.

Commenting on the findings, lead author Judith Moskowitz said: "Even in the midst of this stressful experience of testing positive for HIV, coaching people to feel happy, calm and satisfied – what we call positive affect – appears to influence important health outcomes."

For the study, which was based in San Francisco, 80 participants (primarily men) were taught a set of eight skills over five weekly sessions to help them experience more positive emotions. Another 79 participants were in the control group, meaning they were not taught the skills.

Moskowitz and colleagues designed the tools based on evidence showing these particular skills increase positive emotions. Some of the skills included:

1. Recognising a positive event each day

2. Savouring that positive event and logging it in a journal or telling someone about it

3. Starting a daily gratitude journal

4. Listing a personal strength each day and noting how you used this strength recently

5. Setting an attainable goal each day and noting your progress

6. Reporting a relatively minor stressor each day, then listing ways in which the event can be positively reappraised. This can lead to increased positive affect in the face of stress

7. Understanding small acts of kindness can have a big impact on positive emotion and practising a small act of kindness each day

8. Practising mindfulness with a daily ten-minute breathing exercise, concentrating on the breath.

Fifteen months after the interventions, 91% of the intervention group had a suppressed viral load (meaning less of the HIV virus in their blood) compared to 76% of the control group.

The researchers noted that in addition to the potential benefit of a lower viral load on the infected person, there may be public health benefits.

"From a public health perspective, that is potentially huge for prevention of HIV," Moskowitz said.

"HIV is less likely to be transmitted with a low viral load. To have a difference like that is amazing."

The reduced viral load could be because of a stronger immune system, Moskowitz said, which has previously been linked to positive emotion.

The positive emotion intervention also improved mental health. At baseline, about 17% of the control group and intervention group reported being on antidepressants.

15 months later, the intervention group was still at 17% but the control group's antidepressant use rose to 35%.

"The group that learned coping skills did not increase antidepressant use, whereas overall the control group increased its antidepressant use," Moskowitz said.

In addition, the intervention group was significantly less likely to have repeating, intrusive thoughts about HIV.

The paper was published in the *Journal of Consulting and Clinical Psychology.*

18 April 2017

⇨ The above information is reprinted with kind permission from The Huffington Post UK. Please visit www.huffingtonpost.co.uk for further information.

British scientists may have cured a man of HIV with experimental new therapy

It's very early days, but this experimental therapy could spell the end of the virus.

By Thomas Tamblyn

ritish scientists could be one step closer towards finding a permanent cure for HIV.

A 44-year-old social worker in London appears to be completely free of the virus after undergoing an experimental therapy technique.

The man was first given a vaccine which helped his immune system detect infected cells, and then took Vorinostat, a drug which is normally used in experimental cancer treatment trials.

The Vorinostat then activates dormant infected cells that would normally slip through the net allowing the body's immune system to detect and kill every last infected cell.

In simple terms what this combination of treatments does is remove the camouflage that allows HIV to remain hidden and then shine a spotlight on it allowing the immune system to clearly identify infected cells and kill them.

The researchers have said that there's an extremely long way to go before they start throwing parties. For starters this is just one man in a trial that involves 50 people.

All 50 will need to show similar responses to the treatment, and then even if they do they'll need to be continually tested for the next five years to make sure the virus has been completely eradicated.

That said, this is promising news. For starters this method is essentially a complex and aggressive form of drug therapy, far less invasive and complex as a technique like gene editing.

HIV is a virus which attacks the immune system of the human body, making it harder for us to fight off even the mildest illnesses such as colds or coughs.

There is currently no cure for HIV; however, modern treatments allow those infected with it to go on to live a long and healthy life. AIDS is the final stage of the HIV infection, it occurs when the body can no longer fight life-threatening infections. Those who have been diagnosed with HIV early on will not go on to develop AIDS.

3 October 2016

⇨ The above information is reprinted with kind permission from The Huffington Post UK. Please visit www. huffingtonpost.co.uk for further information.

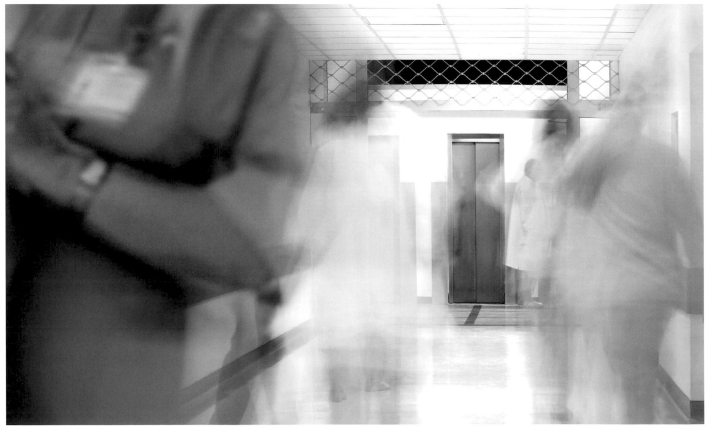

University sells HIV testing kits through vending machines

The move comes as part of efforts to improve HIV prevention in China, where increasing numbers of students are being diagnosed with the virus.

By Rachel Pells

Universities in China are offering students a discreet way to test for HIV using soft drink vending machines.

Students at Harbin Medical University in northern China can purchase HIV self-test kits from the same machines selling cans and instant noodle packs on campus.

The college is the second in Heilongjiang province to install the specialised vending machines after the Harbin University of Science and Technology, local news site Xinhua reported.

The move is part of an HIV prevention initiative by the Chinese Association of STD and HIV/AIDS Prevention and Control (CASAPC), which installed nine of the machines in five universities across China last year.

Students can purchase the test kits for 30 yuan (less than £3.50) – almost ten times less than the average market price in China, where medical care can be costly.

After using the kit to take a urine sample, consumers can drop the samples into a deposit drawer in the specialised machine.

CASAPC staff retrieve the samples from the vending machine, and students can view their test results online anonymously by entering a unique code.

> **"Students at Harbin Medical University in northern China can purchase HIV self-test kits from the same machines selling cans and instant noodle packs on campus"**

Around 654,000 people in China live with HIV or AIDS – a low percentage of the overall population especially when compared to the UK.

Recent figures have highlighted a rise in the number of students contracting the virus, however. Around 2,320 young people aged between 15 and 24 tested positive for HIV or AIDS last year – four times that of six years ago.

The prevalence of other sexually transmitted infections (STIs) is also increasing in the country, a problem some say is in part due to increasing reluctance among young people to use condoms.

People with HIV are often discriminated against in China, with those known to have the virus more likely to lose their jobs, education and healthcare, according to the global HIV charity AVERT.

The number of people taking HIV tests in China rose from 60 million in 2010 to 140 million last year, but fewer than ten students were reported to have purchased tests from the Harbin Medical University since a vending machine was installed in November last year.

"We can't eliminate the virus for now, but at least we can prevent it from spreading," said Wang Mengjiao, a third-year student of Harbin Medical University. "For that purpose, it is important to take part in voluntary testing."

17 April 2017

⇨ The above information is reprinted with kind permission from *The Independent*. Please visit www.independent.co.uk for further information.

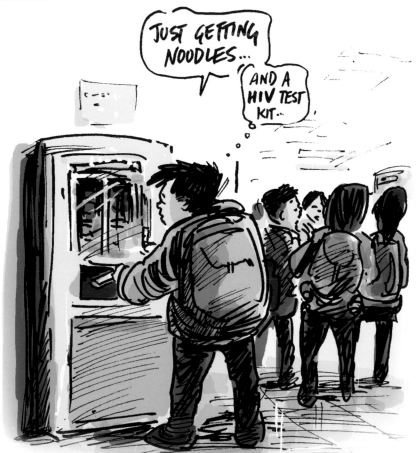

Key facts

⇨ In the 1980s and early 1990s HIV treatment wasn't good at fighting the virus and most people with it were eventually diagnosed with AIDS. But now anti-HIV drugs can control (but not completely get rid of) the virus and far fewer people in Britain develop serious HIV-related illnesses. (page 1)

⇨ Around 101,200 people were living with HIV in the UK at the end of 2015. Of these 101,200, over 13,156 (one in seven) don't know they have HIV because they have never had an HIV test or they got HIV since their last test. (page 1)

⇨ Recent years have seen around 6,000 people test positive for HIV each year – more than half are gay or bisexual men. (page 1)

⇨ Around 47,000 gay or bisexual men and around 49,500 heterosexuals were estimated to be living with HIV in the UK by the end of 2015. (page 1)

⇨ In 2016, 18.2 million [16.1 million–19.0 million] people were accessing antiretroviral therapy. (page 3)

⇨ In 2015, 36.7 million [34.0 million–39.8 million] people globally were living with HIV. (page 3)

⇨ In 2015, 2.1 million [1.8 million–2.4 million] people became newly infected with HIV. (page 3)

⇨ Since 2010 there have been no declines in new HIV infections among adults. (page 3)

⇨ In 2015, 6,095 people were diagnosed with HIV: this represents a new diagnosis rate of 11.4 per 100,000 people. (page 4)

⇨ In 2015, 88,769 people received HIV care in the UK, up 73% from a decade ago (51,449 in 2006). (page 5)

⇨ Despite all the efforts to fight HIV, this year (2015) the European Region has reached over 142,000 new HIV infections, the highest number ever. (page 7)

⇨ Twenty years ago when someone acquired HIV, they would, on average, not live more than 12 years. Today, a young person who becomes infected in the developed world can expect to have a near-normal lifespan with access to lifelong, uninterrupted HIV treatment. (page 8)

⇨ At least 30 countries in the world account for 89% of all new HIV infections. At least 18 of these countries are in Africa. (page 9)

⇨ Sweden has become the first country to achieve the UNAIDS/World Health Organization (WHO) 90-90-90 target, research published in HIV Medicine shows. At the end of 2015, 90% of HIV cases in Sweden were diagnosed, 99.8% of people were linked to care and 95% of people taking antiretrovirals for at least six months had a viral load below 50 copies/ml. (page 10)

⇨ Of the estimated 3.2 million children under the age of 15 living with HIV, approximately 91% reside in sub-Saharan Africa. (page 14)

⇨ Adolescent girls (15–19) account for approximately two thirds of new HIV infections among adolescents. (page 14)

⇨ Only 22% of HIV-positive children in sub-Saharan Africa who need antiretroviral treatment were receiving it in 2013. (page 14)

⇨ Around 2,100 young people and adolescents are infected with HIV every day. In 2013, four million young people aged 15–24 were living with HIV, with 29% aged under 19. (page 15)

⇨ Of all adolescents aged 15-19 who were diagnosed as HIV-positive during 2012, two-thirds were girls. Globally, young girls are more vulnerable to HIV for a number of reasons, but universally the level of HIV knowledge among girls is less than among boys because girls are less likely to attend and finish secondary school. (page 18)

⇨ When Prince Harry took an HIV test live on Facebook, the live streamed event was watched by over two million people. The royal took the test to show how easy it is to be tested. Since then, the demand for at-home HIV test kits has risen 500%. (p.25)

⇨ At the end of 2015 almost half of the estimated 37 million people living with HIV were receiving antiretroviral therapy. Antiretroviral therapies stop the proliferation of HIV in the body to reduce the viral load. This greatly reduces the risk of transmitting the virus to more people. If both sexual partners are receiving antiretroviral therapy then the likelihood of transmission can be reduced by up to 96 per cent. (page 35)

⇨ Scientists have analysed the blood of 170 children from South Africa with HIV who have never had treatment nor developed AIDS. The tests showed that the respondents had tens of thousands of human immunodeficiency viruses in every millilitre of their blood. (page 36)

⇨ Around 654,000 people in China live with HIV or AIDS – a low percentage of the overall population especially when compared to the UK. (page 39)

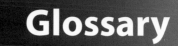

Glossary

90-90-90

A target set by UNAIDS. By 2020, 90% of people living with HIV should know their HIV status, 90% of people diagnosed with HIV will be receiving antiretroviral therapy and 90% of people receiving antiretroviral therapy will have viral suppression.

AIDS

Acquired Immune Deficiency Syndrome. AIDS is a potentially fatal illness. It develops at the most advanced stage of HIV.

Antiretroviral therapy

Drugs that suppress the amount of HIV virus in the body. Antiretrovirals (ARVs) help people with HIV to live relatively healthy lives for a long time, although they do not cure the condition.

Discrimination

Unfair treatment of someone because of the group/class they belong to.

Epidemic

Widespread occurrence of an infectious disease.

Ethnicity

Ethnic origin.

HIV

Human Immunodeficiency. A virus passed-on through certain bodily fluids such as infected blood, genital fluids, breast milk and semen. It cannot be passed through kissing or touching. HIV attacks the cells of the immune system, making it hard for the body to fight infections. Immediately after contracting HIV, a person may experience flu-like symptoms which will then disappear. At later stages of infection, symptoms include fatigue, weight loss, sores in the mouth and pneumonia. HIV can, eventually, progress to AIDS.

Immune system

The immune system is made up of cells, tissue and organs that protect the body from viruses and infections. The HIV virus attacks the immune system and prevents the body from protecting itself.

Prejudice

Referring to prejudgment - forming an opinion before you are fully aware of the facts.

PrEP

Pre-exposure prophylaxis (PrEP) is a pill that people who are at risk of contracting HIV can take daily in order to prevent infection.

Sexually transmitted disease

A disease or infection that is transmitted through the exchange of bodily fluids such as semen or genital fluids.

Stigma

A negative reaction associated with a particular circumstance. Being HIV positive has a `stigma` attached - it often causes others to behave negatively because they are wary of contracting the virus themselves, through touching or close contact, and can invite preconceptions about a person`s sexuality or sexual promiscuity.

Tuberculosis (TB)

A bacterial infection spread through inhaling tiny droplets from the coughs or sneezes of an infected person. This is a serious condition but can be cured with proper treatment. Symptoms include a persistent cough, weight loss, night sweats and high temperature.

Assignments

Brainstorming

⇨ In small groups, discuss what you know about HIV and AIDS.

 • What is the difference between HIV and AIDS?

 • What kind of treatments are available?

 • What is the 90-90-90 target?

Research

⇨ A timeline of HIV/AIDS on page six gives a snapshot of what was happening in regards to HIV and AIDS in 1981 and in 2016. Visit AIDS.gov and look at the whole timeline. Choose a year you find particularly interesting, then choose an incident from that year and do some further research. Create a two-minute PowerPoint presentation to share with your class exploring your chosen incident.

⇨ Research the Terrence Higgins Trust and create a presentation explaining what they do. You could include case studies from people who have been helped by the Trust, examples of their research, etc.

⇨ Sweden is the first country to have achieved their 90-90-90 target. Research how they did this and then look at which countries are struggling to achieve it. Write a bullet point summary of your findings.

Design

⇨ Choose one of the articles from this book and create an illustration that highlights the key themes of the piece.

⇨ Imagine you work for a charity that is campaigning for HIV test-kits to be available in vending machines at universities across the country. Design some posters and a web page that will promote your campaign. You can work in pairs or small groups.

⇨ Design a poster that summarises HIV and AIDS.

⇨ Design a storyboard for a Youtube video which highlights the stigma surrounding HIV. You could choose a setting such as work or school in order to demonstrate your message. If you'd like to take this further and have access to video recording devices, work in small groups and with your teacher to create your video.

⇨ Design a leaflet that will be displayed at your local GP's office, explaining AIDS and HIV, include information about how they are contracted and what treatment is available. You should also provide details of how and where people can be tested.

⇨ Create a campaign that will raise awareness of AIDS and HIV amongst people your age. What kind of campaign would be most successful? Television, radio, web or posters? Produce a campaign plan and include sample designs, scripts or storyboards.

Oral

⇨ Create a PowerPoint presentation that explores the treatments available for those who have HIV. You might also want to look at prevention.

⇨ In small groups, discuss whether you think London should have an AIDS memorial to recognise those who have died from HIV/AIDS.

⇨ As a class, discuss whether home-testing kits for HIV are a good idea. Do you think they would encourage people to get tested?

⇨ In small groups, discuss what you have been taught about AIDS and HIV at school. Create a detailed plan for a lesson that will teach pupils of your age-group about these illnesses. Think carefully about what should be included and consider how you will make the lesson interesting and memorable.

Reading/writing

⇨ Write a one-paragraph definition of the word 'stigma' and then compare it with a classmate's.

⇨ Imagine you are an Agony Aunt/Uncle and have received a letter from someone who thinks they might have HIV but isn't sure how to get tested. Write a helpful response.

⇨ The article on page 32 suggests that "Breaking negative attitudes to women is key to tackling HIV". Write a blog post that summarises the author's opinion and consider whether you agree.

⇨ Choose one of the breakthroughs listed in the article on page 35. Do some more research about it and write a one-page article exploring it further.

⇨ Watch the film *Philadelphia* (1993), starring Tom Hanks. Write a 500-700 word essay answering the following question: 'How does the film Philadelphia (1993) address the social stigma surrounding AIDS and HIV?'

⇨ Imagine that you have recently been diagnosed with HIV. Write a blog post expressing your feelings and thoughts. How do you feel right now? What challenges do you think you will have to overcome? What does the future look like? How will your life change?

Acknowledgements

The publisher is grateful for permission to reproduce the material in this book. While every care has been taken to trace and acknowledge copyright, the publisher tenders its apology for any accidental infringement or where copyright has proved untraceable. The publisher would be pleased to come to a suitable arrangement in any such case with the rightful owner.

Images

All images courtesy of iStock except p.30, 31 SXC and p.36 © Steve Evans. Icon on page 41 © Freepik.

Infographics from Public Health England are reproduced under the Open Government license.

Illustrations

Don Hatcher: pages 8 & 25. Simon Kneebone: pages 16 & 39. Angelo Madrid: pages 3 & 37.

Additional acknowledgements

Editorial on behalf of Independence Educational Publishers by Cara Acred.

With thanks to the Independence team: Mary Chapman, Sandra Dennis, Jackie Staines and Jan Sunderland.

Cara Acred

Cambridge, May 2017